Collaborative Arts-based Research for Social Justice

This book provides a thought-provoking guide to conducting collaborative arts-based research. Focusing on ways that social inquiry might be conducted with marginalised groups to promote social justice, the text offers chapters on:

- telling 'alternative' stories through a variety of methods, from crafts to digital film;
- visual and metaphorical approaches to social research, including photography, art and poetry; and
- performative methods that include drama, dance, music and performance art.

Foster introduces relevant methodological debates, giving a context for understanding when arts-based research can be a fruitful approach to take and outlining a convincing rationale for using the arts as a way of understanding and representing the social world. The book also suggests a range of alternative criteria for evaluating the quality of arts-based research. Illustrative examples from around the world are used throughout the book, and an extended case study is included that focuses on Foster's own collaborative arts-based research.

With their emphasis on the value of participative research and social justice, arts-based methodologies are becoming increasingly popular in health and social research. This is the ideal text for anyone looking to introduce arts-based methods into their research practice.

Victoria Foster is Senior Lecturer in Social Sciences at Edge Hill University, UK.

Routledge Advances in the Medical Humanities

Collaborative Arts-based Research for Social Justice

Victoria Foster

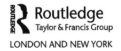

Routledge
Taylor & Francis Group

LONDON AND NEW YORK

First published 2016
by Routledge
2 Park Square, Milton Park, Abingdon, Oxon OX14 4RN

and by Routledge
711 Third Avenue, New York, NY 10017

*Routledge is an imprint of the Taylor & Francis Group,
an informa business*

© 2016 V. Foster

The right of Victoria Foster to be identified as author of this work has
been asserted by her in accordance with sections 77 and 78 of the
Copyright, Designs and Patents Act 1988

All rights reserved. No part of this book may be reprinted or reproduced
or utilized in any form or by any electronic, mechanical, or other means,
now known or hereafter invented, including photocopying and recording,
or in any information storage or retrieval system, without permission in
writing from the publishers.

Trademark notice: Product or corporate names may be trademarks or
registered trademarks, and are used only for identification and explanation
without intent to infringe.

British Library Cataloguing-in-Publication Data
A catalogue record for this book is available from the British Library

Library of Congress Cataloging in Publication Data
Foster, Victoria.
Doing collaborative arts-based research : a guide / Victoria Foster.
pages cm. -- (Routledge advances in the medical humanities)
Includes bibliographical references and index.
1. Arts--Therapeutic use--Research. 2. Art therapy--Methodology. I. Title.
RC489.A72F67 2016
616.89'1656--dc23
2015017274

ISBN: 978-0-415-65692-4 (hbk)
ISBN: 978-0-415-65693-1 (pbk)
ISBN: 978-0-203-07745-0 (ebk)

Typeset in Times
by Saxon Graphics Ltd, Derby

For my father, Robert Foster, and in memory of my mother, Elizabeth Foster

Contents

Figures

Videos

Acknowledgements

I would like to thank all the artists and scholars who have inspired this book. I also wish to acknowledge the women I worked with at the Sure Start programme and the enrichment they have provided, not just to this work, but to my life. I am grateful to Edge Hill University for providing me with the time and resources to complete the book. I would also like to thank friends and colleagues – at Edge Hill University and (much) further afield – in particular, Deirdre Duffy, Kirsty Finn and Peter Kelly, for their thoughtful feedback on various drafts. James Milton has – once again – proved to be both loyal friend and wonderfully diligent reader of the manuscript. Louisa Vahtrick at Routledge has consistently provided advice and support. My father has given me constant encouragement, and has uncomplainingly read draft after draft of the book, whilst my sons, Zach and Otis, have kept up my spirits throughout the process.

1 Introduction

Peeling wallpaper

One of the main strengths of the arts is an ability to provide new perspectives on the lived world, often leading to a 'startling defamiliarisation with the ordinary' (Greene 2000, p. 4). Employed in the research process, the arts enable an examination of the everyday in imaginative ways that draw attention to the cruelties and contradictions inherent in neoliberal society. It is too easy to become inured to our surroundings, to forget how much we *do* know (however partial or limited this knowledge may be) and what our own day-to-day realities tell us about the wider world:

> I put a picture up on a wall. Then I forget there is a wall. I no longer know what there is behind this wall, I no longer know there is a wall, I no longer know this wall is a wall, I no longer know what a wall is. I no longer know that if there weren't any walls, there would be no apartment. The wall is no longer what delimits and defines the place where I live, that which separates it from the other places where other people live, it is nothing more than a support for the picture. But I also forget the picture, I no longer look at it, I no longer know how to look at it. I have put the picture on the wall so as to forget there was a wall, but in forgetting the wall, I forget the picture too …
>
> (Perec 1974/2008, p. 39)

This habituation acts as a barrier in terms of understanding the profound inequalities of the social world and in acting to make positive changes. The minutiae of our lives, even down to our very feelings about them, are continuously being shaped by powerful socio-economic structures. Whilst we remain unquestioning, the 'infinitesimal practices' that 'hegemonic or global forms of power rely on' (Foucault 1980, p. 99) remain unnoticed.

Everyday life is 'marked by difference' (Highmore 2002a, p. 11). There are complex, interconnected ways in which 'discrimination reaches into everyday lives providing a pecking order based on class, "race", gender, age, ethnicity, religion, sexuality, "dis"ability or any other form of difference' (Ledwith and Springett 2010, p. 27). Arts-based research methods enable a diversity of experiences to be communicated in ways that disrupt 'common sense' understandings and act as a reminder that there are possibilities for things to be otherwise. It is here that there are possibilities for small but significant acts of resistance and this enables Susan Finley (2008, p. 72) to proclaim, 'At the heart of arts-based inquiry is a radical, politically grounded statement about social justice'.

The arts also lend themselves to collaborative working and the control participants have over the research process is central to the transformative potential of this methodology. Elliott Eisner (2008a, p. 10), a leading protagonist of arts-based research, describes his vision of a practice that is 'considerably more collaborative, cooperative, multidisciplinary, and multimodal in character'. He continues: 'Knowledge creation is a social affair. The solo producer will no longer be salient'. A collaborative research process offers opportunities to raise critical consciousness, highlight social relations and to promote deeper understanding among participants, facilitators and audiences. This understanding is built on 'emotive, affective experiences, senses, bodies, and imagination and emotion as well as intellect' (Finley 2008, p. 72).

This book explores alternative ways of working with marginalised people to produce knowledge about their lives; knowledge that can draw attention to their lived experience of inequality or stigma and be used to make positive transformations. It advocates a range of arts-based methods to collect, analyse and disseminate data. These methods draw on the literary, visual and performing arts and include storytelling, poetry, crafts, photography, digital technology, collage, short-film making and performance. Such eclectic devices offer ways of 'knowing the self and exploring the world' (Knowles and Thomas 2002, p. 131) in ways that make research accessible outside the academy. This chapter employs a variety of arts-based examples to make a case for the importance of this approach to social inquiry. It then provides a summary of the book and an outline of the forthcoming chapters. The section 'Resistance buried in the everyday' discusses how the everyday, the habitual, can be understood as a source of oppression and also of resistance. A provocative art work provides an illustrative example. The next section, 'Listening with our eyes', explores the need for research practice to attend to the unspoken elements of people's experiences. The arts might enable a move away from a focus on the verbal and the textual, but there is also a requirement to make connections between these personal experiences and wider social relations. The third section, 'Imagining freedom', considers the role of the imagination in research that attempts to promote social justice, and argues that this is intricately entwined with our everyday realities. The act of creatively and collectively exploring our lives enables an acknowledgement that 'Walls protect and walls limit' (Winterson 1985). We need to look beyond them, and doing this in imaginative ways can be subtle, illuminating or even profound. It can 'help us to see the actual world to visualise a fantastic one' (Warner 1995, p. xvi).

Resistance buried in the everyday

There is a significant and fascinating history of studying the everyday (Highmore 2002a; Highmore 2002b; Sheringham 2006). Much of this centres on the French movement of *la vie quotidienne*, which includes the work of sociologists Henri Lefèbvre and Michel de Certeau, the writer Georges Perec and surrealists such as André Breton. Through surrealism, which Highmore (2002a, p. 46) reads as 'a form of social research into everyday life', there is a potential to tap in to 'the unrealized possibilities harboured by the ordinary life we lead rather than rejecting it' (Sheringham 2006, p. 66). Bizarre poetic encounters and strange juxtapositions of everyday objects become 'important artistic strategies that destabilise and cast doubt on the objectivity and conventions of "reality"' (Schulz 2011, p. 14).

One notable interdisciplinary way that this can be seen is through the Mass-Observation project that began in the 1930s in the UK. Founded by Charles Madge, Tom Harrison and Humphrey Jennings, it produced an 'unlikely and disquieting marriage of surrealism and social anthropology' (Highmore 2002a, p. 31). This was an 'anthropology at home' in which members of the public were able to take part. They were recruited and sent out to record their domestic cultures through ethnographic methods of observation and diary-keeping in an arguably 'radically democratic project' (Highmore 2002a, p. 87) that let people 'speak for themselves' (Highmore 2002b, p. 145) and provide a commentary on everyday life with the potential of making changes to it (2002a, p. 111).

In its original manifesto, Mass-Observation produced a list of topics for investigation (Harrison et al. 1937, p. 155, cited in Mengham 2001, p. 28):

> Behaviour at war memorials; Shouts and gestures of motorists; The aspidistra cult; Anthropology of football pools; Bathroom behaviour; Beards, armpits, eyebrows; Anti-semitism; Distribution, diffusion and significance of the dirty joke; Funerals and undertakers; Female taboos about eating; The private lives of midwives.

The 'sheer daftness' of the list is 'in perfect accord with the more facile subversions of surrealist humour' (Mengham 2001, p. 28) but remarkably the idiosyncratic project grew into a well respected enterprise (ibid., p. 27). Through the continuation of the avant-garde practice of making the familiar strange, emerged a 'popular poetry of everyday life' (Highmore 2002a, p. 111) which anticipated the later concerns of reflexive ethnography (Clifford 1988, p. 143) in terms of its preoccupation with multivocality and poetic representations.

In order to attend to issues of social justice there remains a pressing need to view the everyday from an alternative angle, and to 'Tell all the truth but tell it slant' (Emily Dickinson, in Franklin 1998, p. 506). It is through the everyday that the 'endless "quiet" reproduction' of social norms takes place. It is in the everyday that the 'most trenchant ideological beliefs, the most hard-to-fight bigotries' lurk (Highmore 2005, p. 6). Perec's work on the 'infra-ordinary', as well as attending marvellously to the peculiarities of *la vie quotidienne*, highlights the political importance of *questioning* the habitual:

> But that's just it, we're habituated to it. We don't question it, it doesn't question us, it doesn't seem to pose a problem, we live it without thinking, as

if it carried within it neither question nor answers, as if it weren't the bearer of any information. ... In our haste to measure the historic, significant and revelatory, let's not leave aside the essential: the truly intolerable, the truly inadmissible. What is scandalous isn't the pit explosion, it's working in coalmines. 'Social problems' aren't 'a matter of concern' when there's a strike, they are intolerable twenty-four hours out of twenty-four, three hundred and sixty-five days a year.

(Perec 2008, p. 209)

Ideology, or the 'stories a culture tells about itself' (Lather 1991, p. 2), permeate our everyday experiences. These stories are interwoven through our social and cultural lives, their transmittance often unconscious and inarticulate. Terry Eagleton (2007a, p. 114) poses the question of how we combat a power that is 'subtly, pervasively diffused throughout habitual daily practices', power which has become the '"common sense" of a whole social order, rather than one which is widely perceived as alien and oppressive'.

Yet if the everyday is a source of oppression, it is also in the everyday that resistance is embedded, 'buried in everyday activities' (Weitz 2001, p. 667). A recent exhibition at Manchester's Whitworth Art Gallery, 'Walls Are Talking: Wallpaper, Art and Culture', provides a series of potent examples of how the everyday domesticity of wallpaper, this '"merely" decorative ... innocuous backdrop to our lives' whose 'very ubiquity renders it invisible' (Woods 2010, p. 12), can be subverted in order to rupture complacency. The exhibition presents avant-garde work from a range of artists who have produced wallpapers with their own designs, patterns or motifs. Robert Gober's series of installations consists of wallpapers printed with disturbing, provocative images. *Male and Female Genital Wallpaper*, as the title would suggest, comprises recurring images of genitalia (Figure 1.1). They are sketchily drawn and would look more in keeping scratched into the door of a public toilet cubicle than on a vast expanse of wall in the rarified gallery setting. Yet it is precisely this disturbing of context that communicates Gober's message concerning the ways that sex and sexual identity are kept hidden and private. The work was first produced in 1989, at the peak of the AIDS crisis, a time when sexual practices did begin to be discussed more publicly. However, a downside to this was an increased and blatant discrimination of gay men (Saunders 2010, p. 34). The very way that wallpaper envelops the room, and is a constant background to daily life, is an important factor in Gober's work. The use of those troubling images, repeated over and over again draws attention to the ways in which 'social, sexual and political attitudes and codes of behaviour become ingrained by a process of repetition and familiarization so insidious and stealthy that we neither notice nor question them' (Saunders 2010, p. 33).

The consciously political, emancipatory knowledge that this book focuses on draws attention to such 'contradictions distorted or hidden by everyday understandings' (Lather 1991, p. 52) and to the possibilities for social change. Processes of knowledge production do not stand outside ideology, but they do

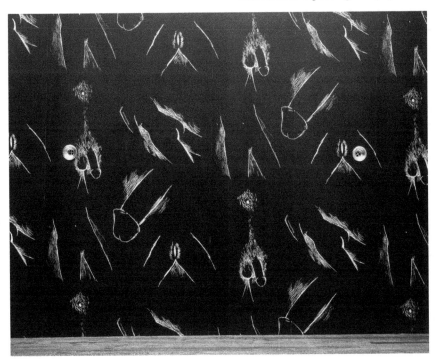

Figure 1.1 Robert Gober, *Male and Female Genital Wallpaper,* 1989, silkscreen on paper, 15' × 27", edition of 100

Source: © Robert Gober, Courtesy Paula Cooper Gallery, New York.

hold potential for challenging the status quo. Such a challenge requires 'a different way of making sense of the world' (Ledwith and Springett 2010, p. 160).

Listening with our eyes

Whilst the collaborative approach suggested in this book draws on the experiential knowledge of the subaltern, there is a tension in terms of assuming people are 'experts in their own lives'. Indeed, Les Back (2007, p. 11) is particularly dismissive of this notion, arguing that the 'up close worlds that people experience combine insight with blindness of comprehension and social deafness'. In *The Art of Listening* (2007), Back calls for a sociology that listens much more vigilantly, but also engages critically with what is being said. Although his methodological approach is quite different from the one outlined here, his work holds much resonance for this book. Back's raw but beautifully nuanced accounts of violence and pain weave together people's stories and images with sociological rigour. The tattooed man lying in a hospital bed, voiceless, dying, the ink telling the story of his journey around the world as a merchant seaman; the brashly styled, 'larger than life' Black woman who calls everyone 'Honey' yet whose confident demeanour hides 'confidential frailties' (ibid., p. 106). A palpable respect is demonstrated for the subjects of his research, and thoughtful links are made between the 'traces that they leave' (ibid., p. 153) and global political forces. Back employs images that are powerful and haunting, images that call for us 'to listen with our eyes' (ibid., p. 100).

Listening is certainly a key element of social justice oriented research, and this is not necessarily an undemanding process, as the Italian philosopher Gemme Corradi Fiumara discusses in *The Other Side of Language* (cited in Kester 2004, p. 107):

> We have little familiarity with what it means to listen, because we are … imbued with a logocentric culture in which the bearers of the word are predominately involved in speaking, molding, informing.

Listening with our eyes requires an attention to nuances, silences, embodied feeling, and also making links with wider social injustices. Purabi Basu's lyrical short story 'French Leave' (also sometimes translated as 'Radha Will Not Cook') addresses the daily chore of cooking which still largely falls to women across much of the globe. It tells of a woman, Radha, who awakens one morning and decides not to cook that day. Her family is horrified when she refuses to provide any meals. Her mother-in-law's ever shriller weeping and wailing is loud enough to attract the neighbours' attention. Rhada's husband shakes her shoulders 'violently' and smashes crockery around her. Radha remains silent and unmoved throughout this cacophony:

> Radha went and quietly sat on the steps leading down to the pond, dipping her feet in the water. Behind her the voices were not merely in chorus; they were shouting the house down.
>
> (Basu 1999, pp. 10–11)

Poetic images abound throughout the story. The natural world surrounding Radha is in rhythm with her rebellion. Flowers toss their heads; little waves break upon the edges of the pond 'in chuckles'. The story closes with Radha gathering her son to her bosom and breastfeeding him. Four-year-old Sadhan is unused to this, as is Radha's body, but before long 'bubbling white milk' is flowing from the child's 'busy lips' and Radha is satisfied with her resolution not to cook.

Swati Ganguly and Sarmistha Dutta Gupta (cited in Singh 2009, p. 2) trace the appeal of the story to 'the subtle way in which such subversive potentials are teased out in a narrative'. Basu's light touch belies the simmering layers of injustice that have led to Radha's subservient position, and the potency of her resistance and transformation. Whilst the body, grounded in everyday life, may be understood as a vehicle for oppression, so can rebellion be seen in Radha's bodily responses to the novel situation she has created. As Simon Williams (1998, p. 438) argues, 'Bodies, in short, from their leaky fluids to their overflowing desires and voracious appetites, are first and foremost transgressive: demonstrating their continual resilience to rational control'.

Madhu Singh (2009, p. 8), drawing on Scott's (1985) work on everyday resistance, acknowledges the power that Radha's silence conjures. Not only is it a 'bold step against social convention', it also highlights the plight of women who are 'obliged to remain silent and suffer without protest'. Silence can be seen as a form of dissent but there is a paradox here, given that there is much emphasis in social justice oriented research on 'giving voice to' the oppressed. Yet the notion of 'giving voice' does *not* mean that everyone has to speak: 'In dialogue one has the right to be silent' (Freire in Ledwith and Springett 2010, p. 135). In fact, it is only through silence, 'when we sit with our unknowing and questioning', that transformation takes place (Ledwith and Springett 2010, p. 155). In terms of participatory practice, Uma Kothari (2001, p. 151) observes that the most subversive move participants can make is through *not* participating: 'exclusion can be empowering and even necessary in order to challenge existing structures of domination and control'.

Whilst it is important to recognise silence as a problematisation of more conventional, rational notions of participation, social change does always imply and require some aspect of conscious and purposive agency in the context of working with others. There are various forms of resistance described in this book. These tend to be small scale and localised, 'centring on the destabilizing of truths, challenging subjectivities and normalizing discourses' (Thomas and Davies 2005, p. 720). Notions of unruly bodies and rebellious or transformative silence also have epistemological relevance. Arts-based ways of knowing can encompass nuanced, tacit and embodied knowledge. Awareness, however, is needed to ensure that the work produced is not as 'exclusionary, monologic, and hegemonic' as that produced by other methods; for Tom Barone (2008, pp. 38–39), the solution lies in challenging the dominant 'master' narrative, but not in producing a totalising counter-narrative. Rather the scope for social justice oriented research comes through 'luring an audience into an appreciation of an array of diverse, complex, nuanced images and partial, local portraits of human growth and possibility'. Through this movement towards greater compassion, Sherry Shapiro (1999, p. 16), in her work on the relationship of dance to social justice issues, senses freedom. This is a relational freedom which opens up 'opportunities for greater human contact and reciprocity … It is a movement grounded in the concrete dance with life'.

Imagining freedom

Wall

I am not hollow.
One tap and I sing like a Tibetan bowl
    soar high as Cassiopeia
    gather harmonics like clouds.
Desert-throated
thick with dirge in my basest of notes
one touch and I am a chorus.

I have become a chain
    linked within the speed of silence
    that reverberates, cone-shaped, through hardness
until I am ringed with hiccups and stutters
    the only sound an 'ah'
    when I open my mouth.
Notes, like thoughts, have trickled out
slithered into drains wet with sludge.

I tiptoe through fragments
in this house of clay
    to find moments of you that are stone:
onyx eggs, I roll them in my hand
    smooth them in the webbing between fingers.
Cool as dawn, I press them against my cheek
    chill the blisters off my skin
where no words have cut through.
Wait for the silence to break.

> (Barbara Marsh 2003, p. 164.
> Reproduced with kind permission from the poet.)

Arts-based methods offer potential for research participants and their audiences to engage the imagination and to produce diverse counter-narratives. The imagination arguably extends the limited possibilities that the didactic mind produces:

> [The imagination] does not engage things in a cold, clear-cut way but always searches for the hidden worlds that wait at the edge of things. The mind tends to see things in a singularly simple, divided way: there is good and bad, ugly and beautiful. The imagination, in contrast, extends a greater hospitality to whatever is awkward, paradoxical or contradictory.
>
> (O'Donohue 2004, p. 138,
> cited in Ledwith 2011, pp. 61–62)

Employing arts-based methods in the process of knowledge production can challenge the binary thinking inherent in much traditional research practice. Dichotomous categories and dualistic thinking – for example, of self/other, empowered/disempowered, male/female – 'leave little room for multiple and sometimes competing realities' (Wahab et al. 2015, p. 10). This is a hierarchical perspective based on superiority/inferiority which lends itself to domination and oppression (Ledwith 2011, p. 39). Arts-based research shuns the 'stability and certainty' that more conventional research strives to attain, favouring 'disequilibrium' (Barone and Eisner 2012, p. 16). There are even possibilities here for our understanding of knowledge to 'sit within a sense of mystery' (Fernandes 2003, p. 99).

As discussed above, the imaginary can assist in highlighting the absurdity of the everyday, and acknowledge if not resist some of its brutality. Within this notion lies the anticipation of a better life: 'A defiant imagination ... defies the constraints of expectation and the everyday ... because the imagination – liberated by engagement with cultural expression – is necessary to the achievement of all we hope for as a society' (Max Wyman, cited in Clover and Stalker 2007, p. 1). However, the imagination is not always a positive, 'superior realm' (Eagleton 2007b, p. 22). Rather, it is 'able to project all sorts of dark, diseased scenarios, along with a number of utopian ones' (ibid., p. 23). Its links with empathy, and feeling one's way into the worlds of others, can also be problematic. Eagleton equates the process of exploring the imaginative worlds of others to that of exploring other cultures; myriad other cultures. Entering others' 'charming' imaginary worlds, whilst holding one's own as the norm ('and thus scarcely a culture at all') smacks of imperialism (2000, p. 46). This is a tension that must be negotiated within a social justice oriented research process, but as Greene (2000, p. 28) acknowledges, 'the role of the imagination is not to resolve, not to point the way, not to improve. It is to awaken, to disclose the ordinarily unseen, unheard, and unexpected'.

Joanna Latimer and Beverley Skeggs (2011, p. 393), in a rather different vein, also argue that the imagination is rooted in socio-political and cultural contexts. In fact, it is 'one of the key sites in which all political and cultural agendas are played out'. This 'sociological imagination' is a new interpretation of C. Wright Mills' (1959) classic work which has long influenced sociology in terms of recognising the relationship between personal experience and wider society. Latimer and Skeggs (2011, p. 394) draw on the strengths of this contribution, but also stress the importance of not privileging any one perspective. Rather than focusing on *the* sociological imagination, they call for an opening up of possibilities. A closure of the imagination would dangerously 'fix the ways in which we think and conduct ourselves and make permanent the endless divisions that rivet the world into place'.

Norman Denzin (2003, p. 226) also acknowledges the difficulty of translating private troubles into public issues – as Wright Mills advocated – in neoliberal societies. He sees the need for a 'critical imagination' that is 'radically democratic, pedagogic and interventionist'. This would challenge racial, sexual and class discrimination in its commitment to transformations of global capital (ibid., p. 227). Denzin's (ibid., p. 226) critical imagination identifies the variety of men, women and children that currently prevail: 'war widows and orphans, Afghan tribal lords, filthy rich CEOs, homeless persons, Texan politicians, Palestinian refugees, militant Islamics, right-wing Christians, white supremacists, skinheads, bisexuals (sic), transgendered persons, gays and lesbians (sic) ...' It is in these multiplicities, this opening up of possibility and location, that the imagination is potentially transformative. Latimer and Skeggs (2011, p. 399) stress the requirement of an 'ethical commitment to keeping open', and they equate Foucault's concept of curiosity with the imagination:

> Curiosity is a vice that has been stigmatized in turn by Christianity, by philosophy and even by a certain conception of science ... I like the word however. To me it suggests something altogether different: it evokes

'concern'; it evokes the care one takes for what exists and could exist; an acute sense of the real which, however, never becomes fixed; a readiness to find our surroundings strange and singular; a certain relentlessness in ridding ourselves of our familiarities and looking at things otherwise; a passion for seizing what is happening now and what is passing away; a lack of respect for traditional hierarchies of the important and the essential.

(Foucault, 1996 [1980], p. 305,
cited in Latimer and Skeggs 2011, p. 399)

The imagination, then, is not something that is opposed to reality. It is entangled with experience, but it is not just about looking inside ourselves. There are possibilities here to work with others to challenge our limited perspectives.

Summary of the book

The book explores the potential for arts-based research to contribute to positive social change. It is argued that all research is a 'profoundly political exercise' (Humphries 2008, p. 1) and thereby holds the dual possibility of maintaining the status quo or posing a challenge to it. 'Arts-based research' is employed in this book as an umbrella term for a number of qualitative approaches to social research that draw on the visual, literary and performing arts. It is intended to cover methodologies that call themselves arts-informed research, A/R/Tography and performative inquiry, among others. Social justice is understood as a plural model which takes into account distributive, cultural and associational notions (Cribb and Gewirtz 2003, pp. 17–18). Thus whilst it stresses the importance of the goal of reducing inequalities of material, social and cultural resources, it also acknowledges difference and diversity, multiplicities of experience, and the concepts of domination and oppression. Moreover, there is a need for participation in decision-making, not least because this acknowledges 'the role of those most disadvantaged by social injustice, as actors – rather than simply victims – in the search for social justice' (Craig 2002, p. 672).

I have chosen to use the term 'collaborative' in the book's title rather than 'participatory' because this is a more encompassing concept. This way of working is not solely about the participation of the researched in the process of knowledge production; it is about teaming up with artists, poets and performers; making links between the academy and communities; and crucially, engaging with audiences. This choice of terminology does not, however, avoid the substantial critique that has been levelled at participative approaches. Grant Kester (2011, pp. 1–2) notes that whilst the primary meaning of collaboration is straightforward ('to work together' or engage in 'united labour'), this is 'shadowed' by a more sinister meaning. Here collaboration is understood as betrayal, 'to cooperate treasonably, as with an enemy occupation force'. Although Kester's focus here is on contemporary global art, it could equally apply to the social research agenda when he makes the observation that this 'ambivalence, the semantic slippage between positive and negative connotations … is fitting'.

The book intends to hark back to Patti Lather's (1991) call to consider ways of connecting research methodology to theoretical concerns and political commitments. There are many possible routes to this end: new, experimental and established paths. The book is designed to encourage readers – academics, practitioners, activists, students or professionals – to develop their own meaningful research practice, whilst openly acknowledging the limits of this practice. Since Lather first raised her challenge there have been significant developments in research methodology and epistemology. Critical and interpretive approaches to knowledge production have been rigorously problematised by postmodern and post-structural thinking, leaving us at a stage of ideas about truth-seeking and representation that is frequently described as 'mess' (Crotty 1998; Law 2004; Lather 2010). Postmodernisms have drawn attention to the partiality of our knowledge and the difficult task of representing it in any meaningful way. Power relations are complex and are inextricably intertwined with processes of knowledge production, and it has been argued that participatory, 'emancipatory' approaches are just as implicated in the exercise of power as any other (Kothari 2001). In the field of social policy as well as health and social care research, ubiquitous 'evidence-based' approaches – that require detached, 'scientific' method – threaten to stifle any alternative. However, drawing on Judith Butler's (1993) work, Lather (2007, p. 37) understands that it is not sufficient to focus on these inadequacies: 'The task is to meet that limit, to open it as the very vitality and force that propels the change to come'.

The examples of work that are discussed in the book cross disciplinary boundaries and are drawn from a variety of different fields in the arts, humanities, social science, social work and health. Whilst many consist of arts-based research projects, others include postmodern ethnographies, contemporary art works and theatre performances. There are also a number of images drawn from literature and poetry which it is hoped will resonate with readers. Here, 'the words mean more than they denote, evoking … other images, memories, things desired, things lost, things never entirely grasped or understood' (Greene 2000, p. 44). These examples enable methodological discussion, highlighting contradictions, weaving 'knowing and not-knowing which is what knowing is' (Spivak 1987, p. 78). They simultaneously explore the ability of the arts to inspire, to educate and illuminate and ultimately they are intended to motivate ideas for new social justice oriented research.

Outline of chapters

Throughout the book there is discussion of various tensions and paradoxes that a collaborative, social justice oriented research approach raises. The current mainstreaming of participatory approaches in health and social care research is acknowledged, and the notion of 'empowerment' and 'emancipation' is challenged. This is important given that the 'rhetoric of empowerment drops on our heads at every turn like confetti' (Dockery 2000, p. 108) and many of the examples of arts-based research – including my own earlier work (e.g. Foster

2007) – claim to empower or emancipate participants without giving sufficient thought as to how this might be the case. This is an ethical issue, although not one that would necessarily concern an ethics committee. The book makes links between social justice oriented research and ethics, arguing that these are inseparable. Whilst particular methods (such as Chapter 4's visual methods) evoke particular concerns in terms of issues of privacy and anonymity, more general ethical issues arise throughout the book. These tend to focus on the extent to which the research practice discussed challenges the status quo and improves lives in the process.

Chapter 2 sketches out some of the theory that underpins the collaborative arts-based methodology advocated in the book. It begins by looking at the current context of research in an era where a 'politics of evidence' dominates. This term is actually oxymoronic, if 'evidence' is to be viewed as set in stone and irrefutable and 'politics' is actively associated with the exercise of power (Denzin and Giardina 2009, p. 12); but its inherent contradiction highlights the pressing need for more research practice that challenges this hegemonic turn in the research field and openly embraces subjectivity, alternative storytelling, metaphor and emotion. The chapter reflects on aspects of critical theory, feminisms and postmodernisms that are relevant to such a practice whose ultimate aim is to further social justice. There is a focus on participatory and dialogic ways of working, given that these are key to the collaborative aspect of the advocated methodology.

Chapters 3, 4 and 5 look in turn at 'Storytelling', 'Image and Metaphor' and 'Performance'. Finley (2008) notes the 'thin lines of epistemological difference' between these forms, and the issues that arise in discussion of particular methods often apply more generally as well. Chapter 3 discusses the human need for stories, drawing on the narrative turn in the social sciences as well as the much older traditions of oral storytelling, folk and fairytale. Arts-based methods offer rich and diverse ways of storytelling, and the chapter looks at a series of projects that involve in turn quilting, beadwork and short film. The extent to which arts-based methods can encourage different and diverse stories to be told and heard is queried. Because stories are understood as artful constructions, the issue arises as to why one story is told rather than another. Some of the factors involved in these constructions are considered, as is the extent of analysis that is required when employing arts-based methods in data collection. The chapter considers 'silent' voices and 'defiant' voices, and asks whether or not an 'authentic' voice can ever be captured. This theme of 'voice' remains important in Chapters 4 and 5.

Chapter 4's focus on image and metaphor involves discussion of the visual turn in the social sciences and the use of metaphor as a way of attempting to capture the spirit of research encounters. The chapter looks at projects that involve participatory photography, collage, poems and an ambitious art installation. Examination of power relations in research remain an important element of this debate. The chapter also introduces other significant themes in arts-based research. These include emotion as a form of knowledge, the aesthetic power of arts-based research, and potential audience reactions. Chapter 5's focus is on performance and it looks at dance, music, performance poetry and drama. It draws from the performative turn in the social sciences and also from applied theatre studies. These are embodied methods and as such there is much consideration given to embodied knowing and to the affective reaction of audiences to performances. Reaching a wide and varied audience is extremely important if research is to effect social change. However, there is a risk of voyeurism inherent in these arts-based performative approaches, and although one of the much vaunted strengths of arts-based methods is to evoke empathy, there are limits to this empathy and these are discussed.

Chapter 6 consists of a case study which describes elements of my own experiences of applying arts-based methods in a collaborative research project with poor working-class women at a Sure Start project in the UK. I employ the notion of the carnivalesque in order to focus on some of the tensions inherent in the methodology. This is hinted at in earlier chapters, which include tropes such as the trickster and images from the circus. The intention with this chapter is to look at how the research methodology worked in practice and the extent to which its successes can be seen as enduring over time. The carnival hinges on the inversion of accepted hierarchies, but this inversion is time-bound:

> An everlasting carnival does not work. ... The essence of the carnival, the festival, the Feast of Fools, is transience. ... Things don't change because a girl puts on trousers or a chap slips on a frock, you know. Masters were masters again the day after Saturnalia ended ... it was back to the old grind.
>
> (Carter 1994, p. 109)

Chapter 7 continues to think about ways of evaluating the success or otherwise of collaborative arts-based research for social justice. This includes a critique of criteria that are often employed in the making of judgements on research. Suggestions for alternative criteria are explored. Aesthetic issues are discussed: the artistic merits of the art work produced, the work's engagement with its audience and whether it successfully offers up an alternative account that challenges the status quo. It is argued that beauty can be understood as a force for good, but this involves moving away from traditional notions of aesthetics. Research for social justice also needs to negotiate issues of commodification, which can be particularly pronounced in the academy. Focusing on process and on embodying the values which we espouse – kindness, tolerance, acceptance of difference – in our everyday interactions is crucial.

This discussion of process is continued in the book's conclusion. Here attention is drawn to the pleasure and enjoyment that can be experienced through a carnivalesque approach to research. Links are made between humour and resistance as the book surmises that meaningful relationships are essential in research for social justice. In so doing, we can find moments of joy in a life that is all too often demanding and bleak.

2 Intellectual acrobatics

Taught only by reality, can reality be changed.

(Brecht 1977, p. 34. From The Measures Taken.
© Brecht Estate, reproduced with permission.)

The title of this chapter refers to issues in doing research in the context of growing neoliberalism, issues of 'intellectual acrobatics' (Jones and Novak 1999, p. 100) that can contribute to oppression and exploitation of 'the researched'. 'Acrobatics', as a metaphor, evokes the circus and the carnival, motifs that crop up throughout the book – and motifs that are, in turn, intended to evoke ambiguities, a sense of being on the margins, and balancing acts as aspects of the research experience. They also suggest the notion of liminal spaces: places of possibility and transition, illusion and paradox.

> He thought of the Indian rope trick, the child shinning up the rope in the Calcutta market and then vanishing clean away; only his forlorn cry floated down from the cloudless sky. How the white-robed crowd roared when the magician's basket started to rock and sway on the ground until the child jumped out of it, all smiles! ... In Kathmandu, he saw the fakir on a bed of nails, all complete, soar up until he was level with the painted demons on the eaves of the wooden houses; what, said the old man, heavily bribed, would be the point of the illusion if it *looked* like an illusion? For ... is not this whole world an illusion? And yet it fools everybody.
>
> (Carter 1985, p. 16)

Angela Carter's words raise questions over what we think we know. Ideally, through the collaborative research process, people are facilitated to construct and use their own knowledge, and are encouraged to '"see through" the ways in which the establishment monopolizes the use of knowledge for the benefit of its members' (Reason 1998, p. 269). Yet is this ever possible? Is one set of illusions simply being replaced by another? A series of methodological and ethical questions are raised in this chapter, facilitated by the work of postmodern and post-structural scholars.

Postmodernism heralded the end of metanarratives as it acknowledged that there are no 'whole' systems or societies, just 'interwoven, interlocking, overlapping networks of social relations which galvanize power and discourses in different directions' (Kemmis 2001, p. 99). If, as Budd Hall (1993, p. xvii, cited in Maguire 2001, p. 62) articulates, participatory approaches to research are 'fundamentally … about the right to speak', then whose voices can be privileged? Who has the right to speak for whom? Who can 'empower' or 'emancipate' the other? How are these voices represented? This 'endeavour to side with the oppressed' runs a risk of becoming a 'university rescue mission of the voiceless' (Visweswaran 1994, p. 69). There is also a danger of 'overemphasizing consensus and unity' through collaborative, social-justice oriented research, 'thus glossing over the ways in which participative research, too, must be recognized as a noninnocent involvement in a noninnocent space' (Wulf-Anderson 2012, p. 564).

Yet postmodern and post-structural approaches can complement critical theories, leading to a deeper understanding of oppression and ideology and means of addressing this (O'Connor and O'Neill 2004). Knowledge is recognised as partial and 'situated' (Haraway 1988), and objectivity and value-neutrality are shunned. This is counter to the current prevalence of evidence-based approaches in health and social care research. The chapter begins by outlining the neoliberal 'backdrop' against which this problematic resurgence of post-positivism, and the following critique, takes place. It argues that the trouble lies in the lack of space given to alternative means of social inquiry. The section 'Critical conversations' provides a summary of critical and feminist approaches to social inquiry. 'Ventriloquism' similarly gives an overview of some of the most useful contributions of postmodernism to research methodology, not least the emphasis on power. The section 'Masks' begins to consider the part the researcher plays in a collaborative process of inquiry and the extent to which this role requires critical reflection.

The chapter then moves on to discuss the importance of dialogic practice. In the Freirean sense of dialogue, there is an explicit political agenda of liberation from oppression (Rule 2004, p. 323): 'Through dialogue, reflecting together on what we know and don't know, we can then act critically to transform reality' (Freire and Shor 1987, p. 99). The Marxist dictum that it is important not just to understand the world but to change it remains as valid as it ever has been. The time is ripe to pursue social justice, promote human dignity and challenge prevailing forms of oppression within a transformative paradigm (Denzin and Giardina 2009, p. 12). In keeping with the book's spirit, the sections 'Mime' and 'Illusions' provide examples from the literary and visual arts to illustrate some of these ideas. The chapter ends with 'Ringmasters', which questions the extent to which participatory approaches to knowledge production can hope to challenge the status quo. *Who is actually setting the agenda?* '[B]eware terminology' warns Tim Prentki (2006, p. 3):

[T]he dominant is always quick to colonise the languages of resistance and separate the signifier from the signified via the relentless hegemonic seductions of its media. That which is called 'dialogue' more often than not is a conversation between the powerful and the powerless – be it a dialogue between the G8 nation and the majority world or a dialogue between teacher and child.

The chapter concludes by arguing that, whilst there is certainly a pressing need for methodologies that 'transcend the limitations and constraints of a lingering politically and racially conservative postpositivism' (Denzin and Giardina 2009, p. 12), it remains important to consider carefully the claims that are made in research for social justice, and the roles of various collaborators.

The backdrop

Over recent years, methodological and epistemological discussion seemed to move on from the quantitative/qualitative binary. Such dualistic thinking has been challenged by third wave feminists and postmodern academics (Wahab et al. 2015), and the emancipatory possibilities for quantitative research have been acknowledged by some (Leotti and Muthanna 2015). However, in this present era of neoliberal hegemony, with its managerial and instrumentalist demands and the emergence of 'gold standard' discourses, 'many researchers have been caught up in paradigm wars we had dared to dream were over' (Lather 2010, p. 2). It is the narrow definition of what counts as 'evidence' that is part of the problem, and the 'hegemonic and dominatory pretensions' of particular accounts of method (Law 2004, p. 4). Denzin and Giardina (2009, p. 12) provide a list of those methods currently jostling for the gold standard award. These include Cochrane reviews, randomised control trials, citation analyses, quantitative metrics and rigorous peer review evaluation scales. 'Neoliberalism LOVES quantitative reductionism' (Lather 2012, p. 1023) and disallows what cannot be counted. Evidence-based practice has a strong hold in the field of health and social care, as well as informing government policy. This was particularly prominent in the UK under the New Labour government (1997–2010) but has now spread further afield to Europe and North America and Australia (e.g. European Commission 2008; Marston and Watts 2003; Haskins and Baron 2011) where, under neoliberalism, we have seen 'abuses of the use of scientific authority in the interests of the state' (Lather 2012, p. 1023).

Ledwith and Springett (2010, p. 99) term this evidence-based approach 'a creeping disease' which does not acknowledge that practice is actually inseparable from knowledge or evidence (ibid., p. 62). One of the main problems with this approach is the lack of attention to context. It is considered a mark of validity if research can be replicated in various situations. Data must be observable or measureable, contexts controlled and complexities reduced. The emphasis on objectivity creates a detached distance between the researcher and subject. Thus structural inequality and power relations are hidden. An examination of political relations is, therefore, a necessary part of the research process (Whitmore 1994, p. 98). Without such, research, if not a replication of society, is then a moralistic statement of what 'should be' (Witkin 2000, p. 207). Descriptions of society are reflections of our culture, our values, beliefs and relationships, and if we neglect the wider societal contexts in the process of knowledge production then taken-for-granted assumptions are not challenged. Social inquiry, whether quantitative or qualitative, is without doubt a *political* process; it can never be about detached truth-seeking, even though claims to notions of objectivity and value neutrality persist. Decisions about the choice of subject matter undertaken, the source of funding, and the methodology employed, are all unavoidably, inevitably political in that they are influenced by relations of power. Research is also political in that 'its findings can be construed as relevant to the making of decisions about the way people live' (Oakley 1992, p. 301).

Knowledge 'is never pristine and odour-free; it is always tainted and sometimes it stinks; it is enfleshed within systems of structure and domination, within criss-crossed vectors of power and asymmetrical relations of privilege' (McLaren 1999, p. xi). The knowledge constructed through social research has the potential to sustain hegemonic depictions of its subjects and add further to oppression, whether this process is conscious or not. Kathleen Lynch (2000, p. 89) is clear that 'research which is not oriented towards transformation effectively reinforces inequality by default'. It can also, through the act of 'owning and controlling ... the stories of oppression', add *further* to this oppression (Lynch 2000, p. 80). Critical social science, feminisms and elements of postmodernism have highlighted the extent to which imperious claims to 'scientific' truth have long perpetuated, if not assisted in creating, social inequality. From the Enlightenment period onwards, the overwhelming emphasis on science and reason 'has disqualified and repressed other ways of knowing that are rooted in embodied experience, orality and local contingencies' (Conquergood 2002, p. 146). Such knowledge is 'constitutive of relations of *ruling* as well as of relations of *knowing*' (Stanley 1990, p. 10). Its powerful discourses ensured that the profession of modern scientific medicine gained its 'hegemonic position' (Abbot and Wallace 1998, p. 19). Positivism also informs the knowledge base of social work (Carey and Foster 2013, p. 255), and thus the profession's present focus on evidence-based practice is not such a departure as it might seem. A backlash against evidence-based approaches is, however, emerging. This can, for instance, be seen in the current, 'eighth moment' of qualitative research (Denzin and Lincoln 2011, p. 3). This moment is concerned with 'moral discourse' and the development of 'sacred textualities'. It calls for '*critical conversations* about democracy, race, gender, class, nation-states, globalization, freedom, and community' (my italics).

Critical conversations

It is recognised within the critical tradition that no research is 'neutral' research. Antonio Gramsci's (1971) theorising has been particularly useful in terms of thinking about how and why inequality becomes the 'default' position. Dominant ideology is so all-encompassing that it is accepted as 'normal' or common sense. Gramsci's interpretation of hegemony 'extends and enriches' this ideology

(Eagleton 2007a, p. 115) through its emphasis on the need to achieve consent from, rather than direct control over, subaltern classes. A ruling power gains consent without struggle, its interests naturally accepted as being in *everyone's* best interests (Brooker 2003, p. 120). Through the process of hegemony the ruling power 'will see its authority reproduced, a subaltern group will aspire to the values and tastes of its superiors, and a "dominated" group will see its lowly status reinforced' (Steve Jones 2006, p. 52). It is such 'common sense' that critical knowledge production needs to challenge. Gramsci's work fell from favour in the 1980s, explains Ledwith (2009, p. 686–687), due to the 'powerful tide of neo-liberalism', along with critiques of metanarratives, with their 'masculinist bias', from postmodernism and feminism. However, Ledwith argues that a feminist, emancipatory praxis owes an immense 'intellectual debt' to Gramsci, not least because it was his concept of hegemony which 'turned the key to the personal as political'.

It was second wave feminism, arising from the women's liberation movement, that challenged the ways knowledge was produced and drew attention to the ways that it excluded women's experiences and maintained existing gender inequalities (Burns and Chantler 2011, p. 7). Consciousness raising was at the heart of this movement, as women began 'to talk together, analyse, and act' in a wide variety of settings, beginning outside the university but soon being accommodated by feminists within the academy (De Vault 1999, p. 26). An attempt was made to provide space for valuing women's lived experiences and giving women a 'voice' in terms of accounts of their lives. Beverley Skeggs (1997, p. 25) highlights the dialectical nature of this process: women's discussions about their experiences enabled new ways of seeing that could be employed to reinterpret previous experiences. Thus experience and interpretation were inseparable. 'Standpoint' approaches best exemplify this process. Sandra Harding (1987) and Dorothy Smith (1987; 1992) were two proponents, albeit rather different in their theorising, of the idea that the particular socially-situated experience of marginalised and silenced groups was a privileged form of knowledge, particularly in terms of challenging oppression. Women's experiences, it was argued, offer potential for 'more complete and less distorted knowledge claims than do men's' (Harding 1987, p. 184). Examining women's everyday worlds (Smith 1987) meant that attention was drawn to personal and intimate aspects as well as to the home, family and housework:

> By locating the politics of gender in the everyday, feminism provoked a transformation of politics itself: who could have predicted that politics would come to include the sexual and the domestic?
>
> (Highmore 2002a, p. 28)

This troubling of everyday experiences is still important in terms of challenging the status quo. Privileging these experiences, however, is no longer unproblematic, either politically or methodologically. Critical inquirers recognise that authentic 'lived' experiences are not untainted; rather in them is 'the voice of an inherited tradition and a prevailing culture' (Crotty 1998, p. 159). Thus they do not speak an objective truth. Moreover, the assumption made by standpoint feminists that a particular position in society provides particular insight brings with it the risk of presenting a 'correct' or authentic version of womanhood and neglecting accounts which are less straightforward to fit into an existing theory or narrative. It is more opportune for some groups to be granted the authority to speak than others, which effectively silences those who do not fit in to current theories or trends. 'This is why' says Skeggs (1997, p. 26), 'experience is such a thorny issue. It marks a space where speaking and silencing are enacted.'

Black and majority world feminists (hooks 1984; Collins 1990; Spivak 1987) were among the first to raise questions of whose voices should be represented; the ways in which these voices should be represented and by whom; and even whether experience itself should be accorded such a central position in terms of building feminist theory (Fonow and Cook 2005, p. 2218). This has led to an expansion of the concept of gender, intersecting it with other societal divisions such as race/ethnicity, class, sexuality and dis/ability on the understanding that identities are multiple and shifting (Byrne and Lentin 2000, p. 8). This focus on intersectionality and the understanding that power relations form a complex web of oppression (Collins 1990) is a useful way of negotiating the 'ambiguity, relativity, fragmentation, particularity and discontinuity' (Crotty 1998, p. 185) that post-modernism has ushered in.

Ventriloquism

Postmodernism and post-structuralism's emphasis on difference and the particular can be seen as conflicting with emancipatory ideals (Humphries 2000, p. 184). In terms of achieving social justice, a degree of unity is necessary, and attending to multiple voices in multiple locations comes with the 'dangerous potential' of fragmentation (Burns and Chantler 2011, p. 71) and summons up 'the specter of relativism' (Greene 2000, p. 156). Postmodernism has thus been met with ambivalence by some feminists and critical researchers. Peter Reason (1998, p. 281), for instance, is troubled by the notion that, in some versions of postmodernism and post-structuralism, voices are 'just voices' with no claim to the truth, 'so the search for voice is seen as being the search for any old voice. And given current power relations on the planet, the first voices likely to be "deconstructed" are those of people already oppressed, the voices of the poor, of women, but also the voices of the body and of the earth itself'.

In terms of furthering social justice, however, postmodernism has usefully taught us that power relationships are ever present on a micro-level in our day-to-day lives. Michel Foucault's theorising, especially his later post-structural work, has been hugely influential in understanding the dynamic nature of power and its indivisibility from knowledge. Rather than viewing power as a top-down force, and something to be possessed, Foucault (1980) considers the complex interplay of mechanisms which create a 'technology of power' (cited in Greene 2000, p. 189), permeating all our interactions. One of the key points that Kothari (2001, p. 141) makes, in an important critique of participatory development discourse, is that '"people's knowledge" or "local knowledge" is seen as a fixed commodity that people intrinsically have or own'. Power is treated as dichotomous – the haves and have-nots. Instead, she argues, 'knowledge is culturally, socially and politically produced and is continuously formulated as a powerful normative construct'.

There is some resonance here with critical thinking, particularly in terms of the potential Foucault identifies for us to be able to 'step back' and to break our 'immersion in the habitual, the everyday' (Greene 2000, p. 189):

> Thought is not what inhabits a certain conduct and gives it its meaning; rather it is what allows one to step back from this way of acting or reacting, to present it to oneself as an object of thought and question it as to its meanings, its conditions, and its goals. Thought is freedom in relation to what one does, the motion by which one detaches oneself from it, establishes it as an object, and reflects on it as a problem.
>
> (Foucault 1984, p. 388, cited in Greene 2000, p. 190)

Greene notes a connection here with Freire's work in terms of relations between thinking and transformative action. Ledwith and Springett (2010, pp. 17–18) also see the value of Freire's work viewed through a postmodern lens, understanding the plurality of oppressions as intersecting forces and appreciating that 'different ways of knowing provide routes to multiple, subordinated truths [which] places us in opposition to the overarching dominant truth embodied in global neoliberalism, a truth that reifies market competition above life itself'. It remains the fact, however, that certain types of knowledge are 'marginalized or suppressed' because they are held by those 'who are themselves socially excluded or adversely affected by unequal power relations' (Smith 2009, p. 75).

The attempt to raise the status of this suppressed knowledge, and increasing awareness in marginalised groups of their potential power, has been troubled in recent years. Lather (2007, p. 15) reflects critically on her own, earlier (1991) work with its pretensions toward 'emancipating' or 'empowering' some others. It is problematic to romanticise subjects and see them as requiring emancipation from 'generalized social oppression via the mediations of liberatory pedagogues capable of exposing the "real" to those caught up in the distorting meaning systems of late capitalism' (ibid., p. 6). Particularly troubling is the notion that critical intellectuals are the solution to the problem of 'the other'. There have even been comparisons drawn between feminist theories and colonial practices in terms of viewing women as needing 'saving' (e.g. Mohanty 1984). Gillies and Alldred (2002, p. 45) are wary of 'simplistic and patronising' claims of 'empowerment' or 'enlightenment' from participatory researchers, not least because a research project is unlikely to directly change the *material* conditions of participants' lives. This may not even be a goal of such practice given that those of 'radically different philosophical and ideological positions', from socialists to neo-conservatives, use the concept of empowerment to advance their positions (Pease 2002, p. 136). The act of inclusion itself, of drawing people in to participate in research, can 'symbolize an exercise of power and control' over them (Kothari 2001, p. 142). The process can also be exploited as a 'technology of legitimation' and, rather than challenging the status quo and professional discourse, may actually be used to support and maintain established ideas (Carr 2004, p. 18). There is certainly a tendency, as Chantal Mouffe (2002, cited in Carr 2007, p. 270) stresses, for a democratic society to want to create 'a rational consensus'. This might involve, metaphorically speaking, 'a tidying up of people's lives' as they 'conform to the boundaries and limitations of the methodological tools' (Kothari 2001, p. 147). This would evidently be 'exclusionary, oppressive and artificial' (Carr 2007, p. 270).

Masks

Various approaches to social research, and feminist approaches in particular, have placed due emphasis on reflexivity in order to make transparent the intentions of the research and to understand how the researcher's subjectivity is inextricably tangled with the lives of research participants (Doucet and Mauthner 2006, p. 41). In more recent years, this practice has incorporated the ways in which researchers 'consciously write themselves into the text', as well as the acknowledgement of audiences' unpredictable reactions to these texts (Fonow and Cook 2005, p. 2219). Indeed, many of the arts-based research projects discussed in forthcoming chapters of the book recognise and integrate these ideas. This can be a worthwhile practice, but it does not necessarily evade those issues of power and control that might still lurk behind it. For instance, too much spotlight on the researcher's position can detract from the subjects of research. In this sense an irony can be detected in the practice of Western feminist researchers putting themselves centre stage when they are engaged in dialogues about decentering the West and giving voice to the majority world (Doucet and Mauthner 2006, p. 42). Focus on reflexive textual strategies can also become solipsistic. Lather (2007, p. 17) draws on Nietzsche's thesis that 'every word is also a hiding place' in order to trouble the notion of reflexivity. For Lather, openness, or 'nakedness', is not about presenting oneself as 'transparent, vulnerable and absolutely frank'. Such 'apparent nakedness', she argues 'is but a mask that conceals a will to power'. This notion of deception is particularly problematic in research that claims to be emancipatory, and in practice that aims to develop close relationships with research participants, for it is here that risks of manipulation and betrayal take on a particularly, personally and socially, potent dimension (Stacey 1988).

The way forward is, as Lather (2007, p. 17) – influenced by Nietzsche – suggests, 'to multiply perspectives towards an affirmation of life as a means to knowledge without guarantee'. This requires accepting uncertainty and rejecting the notion of 'absolute knowledge'. It is from this stance that we need to explore the diverse masks we wear and the roles that we play both in research practice and our wider lives. Surely 'we enact seemingly abstract concepts such as justice, structural oppression, social change and transformation in every moment of our lives, in every relationship, from the most mundane interactions we engage in with strangers in supermarkets to the most intimate relationships we have with loved ones to the most public interactions we have in work, school, society, the world' (Fernandes 2003, p. 19). There is thus a greater profundity inherent in the feminist slogan 'the personal is political' than is sometimes acknowledged (ibid., p. 55). Our interactions are rarely straightforward, though, in any sphere of life. Kamala Visweswaran (1994, p. 100) draws on Bohannon's notion of ethnographer as trickster in her anthropological novel *Return to Laughter*. Visweswaran tweaks this in order to provide a definition of feminist ethnographer as trickster: 'one who does not profess faith in what she believes'. Visweswaran's notion of feminist trickster 'hinges on the supposition that we can "give voice" and the knowledge that we can never fully' do so:

> This requires a trickster figure who 'trips' on, but is not tripped up by, the seductions of a feminism that promises what it may never deliver: full representation on the one hand, and full comprehension on the other. In this scenario, the feminist as trickster mediates between cognitive failure and its success; it is trickster agency that makes the distinction between success and failure indeterminate, alerting us to the 'possibilities of failure'.

The trickster figure is thus one that crosses boundaries, one that confuses divisions: 'Where someone's sense of honourable behaviour has left him unable to act, trickster will appear to suggest an amoral reaction, something right/wrong to get life going again' (Hyde 2008, p. 7). As Prentki (2012, p. 4) observes, 'getting life going again' is one of the trickster's key functions, as he/she is never stagnant, always searching for new ways of doing things. These ways often involve imagination and play, which makes the figure of trickster an apt one for the realm of arts-based research.

There is also certainly an argument for not being stymied by the above critiques. Inaction is not the answer to the political and methodological conundrums that we face. Arthur Frank (2010, p. 73) stresses such a need for movement within research methodology which has a propensity to be turgid and static. Thought 'moves in dialogue', and it is through participating in dialogue that research participants are given opportunities to challenge researchers' – and society's – presumptions. In his work on the trickster, Lewis Hyde (2008, p. 14) aims to 'hold trickster stories up against specific cases of the imagination in action' with the intention that the one will illuminate the other. Should this aim be successful, though, it is not because any truth has been discovered, but rather that 'fruitful coincidences' have occurred. This gentle mockery of discourses of truth suggests that it is the trickster who might playfully take the myth of evidence-based practice apart.

Mime

The Italian novelist and fabulist Italo Calvino recognised the ever-present dialectic between fantasy and reality (Canepa 2008, p. 156). For this reason alone his work has much resonance for this book and its emphasis on exploring the imaginary and the fantastic to draw attention to everyday actualities. 'I am accustomed to consider literature a search for knowledge', he declared (1992, p. 26, cited in Warner 1995, p. ix); and this is certainly evident in his poetic novel *Invisible Cities* (1997), which takes the form of a series of eighteen dialogues between the explorer Marco Polo and Kublai Khan, whereby Polo describes a series of marvellous cities he has visited. One consists only of plumbing: forests of pipe and porcelain bathtubs or lavabos 'like late fruit still hanging from the boughs' (p. 49). Another extravagantly renews itself every day: the people wear new clothes, use new toiletries and new crockery on a daily basis; street cleaners are 'welcomed like angels, and their task of removing the residue of yesterday's existence is surrounded by a respectful silence' (p. 114).

The Khan comes to the slow realisation that all the cities are somehow based on Polo's Venice, yet despite not necessarily believing everything Marco Polo says, he does 'continue listening to the young Venetian with greater attention and curiosity than he shows any other messenger or explorer of his' (p. 5). Indeed he has much to gain from their interactions. Through their dialogue is conjured up some remarkable insight into the city. In spite of the absurdity of the illogical cities that Polo evokes, the Khan is able to discern some nugget of insight, 'the tracery of a pattern so subtle it could escape the termite's gnawing' (p. 6). There is pleasure in gaining this knowledge, as there is a pleasure in listening to Polo's beautifully crafted stories with their startling and moving imagery. There does not necessarily need to be complete trust, or the removal of masks, for something worthwhile to be gleaned. For the reader too – 'the *attentive* reader' (Becker 2007, p. 283; my italics) – the dialogue is delightful and astute. Becker discusses how the novel provides us with sociological knowledge of the city. Through Polo and the Khan's dialogue we come to understand the two men's different positions and the advantages and disadvantages of each. Whereas 'undialogized language is authoritative or absolute' (Bakhtin 1984), there is an indeterminacy here in which 'alternatives are considered, weighed, tried out, rejected, surpassed, returned to' (Becker 2007, p. 274).

This communication is not always verbal. It might take the form of 'gestures, facial expressions, postures, the whole array of body language' in dialogue. A person participates in this dialogue 'wholly and throughout his whole life: with his eyes, lips, hands, soul, spirit, with his whole body and deeds' (Bakhtin 1984, p. 293). It is thus a significant oversight by dominant epistemologies to neglect this 'whole realm of complex, finely nuanced meaning that is embodied, tacit, intoned, gestured, improvised, coexperienced, covert' (Conquergood 2002, p. 146). Methods of knowledge production need to be attuned to meanings that are 'masked, camouflaged, indirect, embedded, or hidden in context' (ibid). This is where arts-based research can prove indispensable, because it provides possible routes of accessing such intangibilities. Arts-based research also highlights the embodied nature of knowing, particularly through the use of performative methods that communicate messages from and of the body. Dialogue 'begins in bodies before it is expressed in symbols, and it returns to bodies once those symbols are expressed. ... Dialogical listening is a responsive act of grasping with one's body' (Frank 2012, p. 40).

Invisible Cities exemplifies these ideas through the fantastical methods of communication that Marco Polo and Kublai Khan devise. Initially the men are without a shared language. Polo could only express himself through gestures, 'leaps, cries of wonder and of horror, animal barkings or hootings, or with objects he took from his knapsacks – ostrich plumes, pea-shooters, quartzes – which he arranged in front of him like chessmen' (Calvino 1997, p. 21). Kublai was forced to interpret these 'improvised pantomimes'. Gradually, Polo not only learns the Tartar language, but also its idioms and dialects – so that he is able to communicate 'the most precise and detailed' accounts. Yet the Great Khan found that each piece of information recalled 'that first gesture or object with which Marco had designated the place' (p. 22) and he gradually begins to lose interest in Marco Polo's words. So too do words begin to fail Marco Polo, until 'little by little, he went back to relying on gestures, grimaces, glances' (p. 39). So a 'new kind of dialogue was established: the Great Khan's white hands, heavy with rings, answered with stately movements the sinewy, agile hands of the merchant'. Nor was the pleasure of this form of dialogue to last; eventually both remained 'silent and immobile' much of the time (p. 39).

With Bakhtin's emphasis on embodiment and also his attention to multiple voices or 'multivocality' in literature, it is not surprising that Pechey (2007, p. 15) sees him as a forerunner of post-structuralism, albeit more politicised. Dialogue for Bakhtin is not only ontological (the way we are constituted) but also ethical (the way we should be) (Rule 2011, p. 929). Kester (2004, p. 119), however, observes that for Bakhtin, the ultimate goal of the interaction is 'the expansion of the authoring subject, for whom the other remains a mere vehicle'. Danow (1995, p. 76) argues that in this context, 'the word of the other serves to define the (essentially absent) word of the self – where the self is the modern *arriviste* and the other is the indigenous native, whose word is his myth and his faith'. It is important to acknowledge these tensions, particularly applied to the notion of the authoritative researcher who often has the last word in accounts of research, and arguably has more to gain from the research process than participants (certainly materially in terms of salary and career prospects). Collaborative arts-based research practice does not escape this bind. Yet, even knowing that the 'dialogical hope of "speaking with"' (Visweswaran 1994, p. 100) may not be entirely realisable, it remains a worthwhile goal.

Illusions

'Dialogical hope' is a substantive feature of new art movements, and there are lessons here for arts-based research. This is art which takes 'a stance for social justice and equality in and with aesthetic in(ter)ventions in the public territory' (Mey 2010, p. 333). Grant Kester's *Conversation Pieces* (2004) details this trend. Based on Bakhtin's notion of art as a kind of conversation, dialogic art is a collaborative process. Kester (2004, p. 10) describes the extent to which this differs from object-based art work which is produced by the artist and subsequently offered to the viewer. Dialogical projects 'unfold through a process of performative interaction'. This is different from public art or community art whereby dialogue may occur prior to production or as a consequence of the art. In the new genre, 'dialogue and production are essentially one and the same and must function as such' (Richardson 2010, p. 20). The work has its roots in the feminist art of the 1970s, particularly Suzanne Lacy's work which understood that 'the separation of artist from society neutralized the impact of art' (Roth 2010, p. xxi). In recent times there has been a renewed desire for collectivity as opposed to the individualism which has become synonymous with neoliberalism (Bishop 2012). Moreover, 'traditional art materials of marble, canvas, or pigment' have been 'replaced by "sociopolitical relations"' (Kester 2004, p. 3).

Dialogical art is often difficult to distinguish from political or social activism (Kester 2004, p. 11). Mel Gray and Leanne Schubert (2010, p. 2316) draw parallels between this kind of art practice and social work. Social workers frequently see their work as a creative endeavour, whereas artists working in this vein are sometimes criticised for being 'like social workers'. This is one reason why Claire Bishop remains sceptical of the dialogical turn and its 'ethics of authorial renunciation' (Bishop 2006, p. 178). Kester (2004, pp. 2–3) is more optimistic in his assessment, and suggests a shift in the way such projects are understood. He describes one such project in which 'the aesthetic experience can challenge conventional perceptions ... and systems of knowledge'. This was conducted by an Austrian art collective, WochenKlausur, in Zurich, and involved bringing together a host of politicians, journalists, sex workers and activists on a pleasure boat on Lake Zurich. As the boat cruised the lake, a series of conversations took place about drug use and prostitution, and the dire situations that the practically homeless sex workers were experiencing due to stigma, violence from clients and harassment from police. From these talks arose a positive intervention consisting of the establishment of a *pension* (boarding house) that provided a safe place for drug-using sex workers to shelter. Interestingly, WochenKlausur is insistent that its work, its 'interventions', be defined as art rather than social work or activism (Kester 2004, p. 101). Founding member Zinggl declares that:

> Art lets us think in uncommon ways, outside of the narrow thinking of the culture of specialization and outside of the hierarchies we are pressed into when we are employed in an institution, a social organization, or a political party.
>
> (cited in Kester 2004, p. 101)

Again, though, the use of art and aesthetic mechanisms does not necessarily mitigate the power relations which can even infiltrate progressive movements and political activist organisations. These operate 'with their own internal investments of power that can transform activism into yet another form of social capital' (Fernandes 2003, p. 56). In fact, the arts and culture themselves, 'and the new patterns of freelance work and self-employment associated with being an artist', have actually become models for a new process of economic growth (McRobbie 2001, p. 1). McRobbie is discussing the UK New Labour government's neoliberalisation of the cultural economy. 'Everyone is creative', a 2001 green paper suggested, but such focus on creativity is not about realising authentic human potential, greater social happiness or imagining utopian alternatives (Bishop 2012, p. 15). It is about good business, increasing employability, reducing crime (Bishop 2012, p. 13). What is particularly interesting is the fact that the rhetoric surrounding this government focus on the arts is indistinguishable from that of practitioners of socially engaged art (Bishop 2012, p. 13).

Helen Nicholson (2005, p. 49) notes the use of techniques derived from the work of Augusto Boal by a British drama company that specialises in corporate work. Whereas Boalian theatre has been built on the Freirean tradition of social transformation, its methods have been put to use in this context with the aim of increasing productivity rather than addressing the moral or political reasons for improving working life. In one sense this mainstreaming of radical ideas is nothing new. For instance, Miwon Kwon (2004, p. 1) reflects on the ways in which 'van-guardist, socially conscious, and politically committed art practices always become domesticated by their assimilation into the dominant culture'. However, the dominance of 'new liberal speak' (Bourdieu and Waquant 2001) is particularly remarkable, particularly in terms of its 'hijacking a language of liberation' (Ledwith 2001, p. 171). The dilution of radical traditions has contributed to neoliberalism's success in diverting attention from an agenda that, through maintaining the politics of a free market, embraces unquestioningly capitalism and globalisation (Jones and Novak 1999, p. 181). It glosses over the fact that this framework is 'one which itself excludes the possibility of an equal society' (Levitas 2005, p. 188). This is markedly the case in the UK at the time of writing, where David Cameron's Conservative/Liberal Democrat coalition government has been in power since 2010. Its emphasis on 'Big Society', encouraging small groups and charities to play a part in providing welfare whilst it continues to dismantle the welfare state, suggests that 'the neoliberal idea of community does not seek to build social relations, but rather to erode them' (Bishop 2012, p. 14). Arts-based research need not play into the hands of the establishment, but it does require careful and critical thinking to avoid doing so. Otherwise, social justice goals are perhaps no more than illusion.

Ringmasters

The collaborative dimension of the research methodology advocated in the book should be open to a similar level of scrutiny. The previous section discussed the relationship of 'radical' arts initiatives to the 'mainstream'. Here the focus is on the fashion over recent years for involving 'non-experts' in shaping UK public and social policy decision-making and research practice, particularly in the spheres of health and social care (Beresford 2002). More recently the spotlight of user involvement has been on research and evaluation processes to the extent that in the case of health and social care research, service user participation can even be a *requirement* of gaining funding (McLaughlin 2006; Cook 2012). Once again this suggests a mainstreaming of radical approaches, this time in terms of mechanisms of knowledge production which set out to emancipate marginalised groups. Worthwhile goals of transformation are reduced to the more humble ones of improved service delivery (Ledwith and Springett 2010, p. 17). This, the authors point out, does 'not change the structures of injustice' that render disadvantaged research participants poor in the first place (ibid., p. 36). There is also a real risk that 'we are complicit, that our practice is reinforcing the very structures of injustice that we claim to transform'. Academics – or social workers, teachers, health care professionals or other practitioners – are no more likely to be enlightened than anyone else, particularly in terms of their relationship to 'an ideological state apparatus and exploitative materialist Capitalist society' (Carey 2011, p. 231). Indeed, their role and status means that they are inclined to be 'more ideologically impregnated'. Carey (2013, p. 209) is concerned that the participation agenda is yet another way of transmitting hegemonic values. He sees this as particularly troubling in the sphere of social work. He asks what the ethical implications are should vulnerable people who might be 'past victims of control-related interventions or poor services', be compelled to engage in 'processes that may further promote such outcomes'.

The emphasis on service user participation in research does, however, conveniently open doors in terms of funding opportunities for research that involves service users or members of the public. My own research at a Sure Start programme in northwest England was successful in receiving two rounds of generous funding, not least because of the political expediency of involving service users in each stage of the research process. I employed the language of 'social capital' and 'cultural capital' in the research proposals, despite being committed to a practice that did not see people's lives as a commodity. I have also implemented participatory approaches in NIHR-funded health research (see Foster and Young 2012), again mindful of wanting to make positive transformations whilst simultaneously being aware of some of the limitations of doing so (Foster and Young 2015).

David Pariser (2009, p. 2), in his rather damning critique of arts-based research, points out what he sees as the 'ultimate irony' of this practice: 'that although arts-based research is supposed to question the standard scholarly research practice of the academy, it originated in that very same academy'. This raises a series of tensions, but again these are not straightforward and they require a tightrope-walk of careful negotiations and compromises. The academy can be restrictive, but it can also open up possibilities and it is not sufficient to accept either position unquestioningly.

Much participatory research began outside the confines of the university, as Budd Hall (2001, p. 171) points out. He considers whether or not universities ought to be involved in participatory research, namely because of the different uses of knowledge in the academy from those in community or workplace situations. Within the confines of the university, knowledge 'is the very means of exchange for the academic political economy' (Hall 2001, p. 176). Yet a participatory approach dictates that 'the knowledge generated, whether of localized application or larger theoretical value, is linked in some ways with shifts of power or structural changes'. It is certainly problematic that community knowledge and practice is not recognised as 'legitimate' by the academy 'until it turns up in the scholarly literature' (DeFilippis 2015, p. 47). Tina Cook (2012) takes issue with the Research Excellence Framework (REF) in the UK. This is a mechanism of assessing the quality and rigour of academic work. Similar exercises take place elsewhere: in the USA for instance, this audit discourse is known as Scientifically Based Research (SBR) or Scientific Inquiry in Education (SIE); in Australia there is a Research Quality Framework (RQF) (see Denzin and Giardina 2009, p. 16). The REF places value on contributions to academic journals which, as Cook (2012) observes, is not necessarily in the interests of those working in communities and employing more accessible and collaborative methods of dissemination such as performance, visual images or an article in a magazine that would reach a wider readership than an academic journal.

Successful collaborative working, however, should mean that there is scope to disseminate findings in a variety of arenas in different ways. Working with a range of practitioners and participants means that workloads are shared and energy and ideas are plentiful. This can also 'maximize the aesthetic qualities and authenticity of the work' which, in turn, will increase the likelihood of it reaching its audience in the intended ways (Leavy 2009, p. 18). The involvement of academics in a community research project can also add kudos to the work. Moreover, there is also an important place for theorising in research practice that aims to further social justice. Although wary of the elitism of academia and the dense inaccessibility of much academic writing, Yasmin Gunaratnam (2009) acknowledges that there remains a 'transformative potential and power' of ideas and theory generated by academics. This is certainly a possibility in arts-based research where the researcher's role might be understood as that of facilitator or a '"liminal servant" whose responsibility is the creation of entrances to emotional, spiritual and ephemeral spaces' (Finley 2008, p. 73). The facilitator provides tools and opportunities for people 'to perform inquiry, reflect on their performances, and preserve, create, and rewrite culture in dynamic indigenous spaces' (ibid., p. 74). This requires acknowledgement of the relational, political and epistemological challenges that any such practice is bound to raise. Romanie van Son (2000, p. 230), for instance, describes her experiences of acting as researcher and facilitator in an arts-based project as being a 'real balancing act and sometimes frustrating'. She frequently had to resist the urge to 'jump in' when the project's pace slowed down or took an unexpected – and less than desirable – direction. At the same time, there *was* a need to maintain a sense of purpose and structure in the process. Van Son (ibid., p. 229) recognises the need for all involved in the project to recognise the 'many different sides' of one another. In this sense, she could be seen to require a variety of 'masks' that included ones which were worn during the games and role plays she took part in together with the women. An aim of these games was to raise everyone's energy levels, van Son's included. At other times, masks might be needed to represent the *differences* between van Son and the participants, not least in terms of social status. Working together can be productive and life-enhancing for researchers and participants, but dissimilarities remain that no research practice can diminish.

Conclusion

The series of conundrums that have been raised in this chapter are returned to throughout the book, all the time bearing in mind that these are not meant to stifle the progress of new ways of collaborative, 'emancipatory' practice, but to keep conversations flowing, even if these conversations include acknowledgement of dilemmas and pitfalls:

> Put all your ideas on one side of the balance, then put everything that negates them on the other, and then you'll be closer to the truth!!!
>
> (Fuentes 1992, p. 230)

Success and failure should be held in tension (Visweswaran 1994, p. 100), and this enables us to 'question the authority of the investigating subject without paralyzing her, persistently transforming conditions of impossibility into possibility' (Spivak, cited in Visweswaran 1994, p. 100). Even Kothari's (2001, p. 152) rigorous critique of participatory research approaches ends on a positive note. She acknowledges the potential for reflexivity and subversion within the methodology and, drawing on Erving Goffman's theorising, recognises 'the possibility that the performer may delude the audience'. Knowledge, as Foucault reminds us, can be used to discipline or emancipate. There remains a potential for freedom, and given that individuals are active agents they 'have the capacity to fashion their own existence autonomously' (Kothari 2001, p. 151).

Critical dialogue can facilitate this emancipatory possibility as it challenges assumptions and values and the habitual ways we think and act. Arthur Frank (2010, p. 73) discusses how 'critical thought can appreciate how expert people are about their own lives while examining ways in which any person's or group's self-awareness is limited'. Sheila Preston (2009b, p. 304), drawing on Freire's work, discusses the counter-project of the transformative vision. Transformations may happen on a local level, not because one party assumes the power to transform the other, but where 'a climate of dialogue and reciprocity enables people to realise their capacity to discover their own transformative possibilities'. Postmodernist thinking is useful to a collaborative arts-based enterprise, particularly in terms of its rejection of universal truths, and the attention it pays to representations of the social world. However, whilst there are 'clear shifts and transformations' taking place, there are also continuities that need to be acknowledged: 'inequalities of social class, race and gender embedded within patriarchy, racist ideologies and hegemonic heterosexuality' (O'Neill et al. 2002,

p. 78). There is a tension involved in appealing to a metanarrative of emancipation whilst retaining a concern with the particular and the local (Humphries 2000, p. 187). This is highlighted in the current neoliberal climate where 'evidence-based' approaches to knowledge dominate, and the language of emancipation has been diluted. The next three chapters explore a host of arts-based projects and question the potential of these methods of research for subversion.

3   Storytelling

'Lor' love you, sir!' Fevvers sang out in a voice that clanged like dustbin lids. 'As to my place of birth, why, I first saw light of day right here in smoky old London, didn't I! Not billed the "Cockney Venus", for nothing, sir, though they could just as well 'ave called me "Helen of the High Wire", due to the unusual circumstances in which I come ashore – for I never docked via what you might call the *normal channels*, sir, oh, dear me, no; but, just like Helen of Troy, was *hatched*.

'Hatched out of a bloody great egg while Bow Bells rang, as ever is!'

The blonde guffawed uproariously, slapped the marbly thigh on which her wrap fell open and flashed a pair of vast, blue, indecorous eyes at the young reporter with his open notebook as if to dare him: 'Believe it or not!' Then she spun round on her swivelling dressing-stool – it was a plush-topped, backless piano stool, lifted from the rehearsal room – and confronted herself with a grin in the mirror as she ripped six inches of false lash from her left eyelid with a small, explosive, rasping sound.

Fevvers, the most famous *aerialiste* of the day; her slogan, 'Is she fact or is she fiction?' And she didn't let you forget it for a minute; this query, in the French language, in foot-high letters, blazed forth from a wall-sized poster, souvenir of her Parisian triumphs, dominating her London dressing-room.

(Angela Carter 1985, p. 7)

Carter's bawdy and irreverent character of Fevvers, performer, trapeze artist, aerialiste, trickster, acts as a reminder that things are not always as they seem. In this opening scene of the novel, she draws the unsuspecting journalist Walser into her fantastical life story, the central premise of which is her claim to have sprouted wings. Fevvers' storytelling is regularly punctuated by Big Ben striking midnight in a disorienting play on temporality. As Carter has declared elsewhere, 'a good writer can make you believe time stands still'. There is also a timelessness to storytelling as a social practice more generally, as shifting versions of tales are handed down through generations and their telling plays its 'primary role ... in the household of humanity' (Benjamin 1969/2006, p. 373). In relation to ethnography, story can be understood to have an enduring quality. Whilst theories become stale, the stories – or 'fictions' given that they are constructed by the ethnographer - that are chronicled in that historical moment of time live on and continue to have much to say (Behar 2003, p. 19). In the same way, literature stands outside the 'tides of scientific "progress" and enlightenment' (Winterson 1996, p. 166). The emotional reality captured by literature is not regarded as progress from dark to light, 'but as a communication with ourselves and across time' and thus it remains fresh and meaningful.

Every 'real' story contains something useful (Benjamin 1969/2006, p. 364), yielding its harvest in corn and gold after being stroked smooth and combed through (Warner 1995, p. 25). The narrative turn in the social sciences has, over the past three decades, recognised stories' function in terms of informing human life. Stories inform not only in terms of providing information, but also because they *give* form to the mess and confusion of life: 'temporal and spatial orientation, coherence, meaning, and especially boundaries' (Frank 2010, p. 2). Frank has contributed to a raft of work on illness narratives (e.g. Frank 1995; see also Hawkins 1998; Mattingly and Garro 2000). These are 'knowledgeable narratives' (Popay et al. 2003) that give alternative accounts of experiences of health conditions to those of health professionals. Social movements also rely on stories that are told within their communities. For instance, Ken Plummer (1995, p. 145) reflects on how, without gay and lesbian stories, 'the gay and lesbian movement may not have flourished'. Indigenous research thrives on story (Tuhiwai Smith 2012). Story enables the handing-down of tribal values based on ancient knowledges (Kovach 2009) and complements the indigenous oral tradition (Archibald 2008).

In her introduction to her volume on fairytales, Marina Warner (1995, p. xii) describes the world of opportunities and thrilling promise that these stories offer, not only in the dark dream realm of fairyland, but in this world too. They suggest the possibility of change, and might 'remake the world in the image of desire'. The extent to which stories can be told, and heard, that challenge hegemonic understandings – those ideas that are so deeply embedded that they seem entirely natural and unquestionable – and offer alternative truths is explored through this chapter. There is a necessity to describe the world 'in ways that make possible encounter with mystery' (Starhawk 1987, p. 26). Viewing the world through this lens means that 'the old systems and structures may themselves be revealed as distortions'. The chapter looks at examples of storytelling through a range of arts-based methods, from traditional crafts through to digital technology in an exploration of the promise they hold in terms of research for social justice. This discussion is woven through with glimpses of the 'magic' and mystery that arts-based research comes close to touching.

Jennifer Eisenhauer (2012, p. 9) reflects on the questions that are possible to ask within the 'juncture' or 'seam' that is created when arts-based inquiry is accepted as research and placed alongside more conventional research 'that relies on linear narratives most often devoid of visual imagery'. These include: What does it mean for something to be research? What are the goals of research? How does the form that research takes impact on what it can achieve? For Maggie O'Neill (2008), it is within this space that transformation is possible. It is here that the imagination can do its work (Greene 2000) and we can reclaim the 'endearing, enchanting, graceful aspects of human existence' (Szakolczai 2007, p. 1), the 'sheer magic' whose visibility has receded through the march of the modern world. Szakolczai's reference to magic is not about supernatural forces (ibid., p. 3). Rather it is 'the possibility to influence the way in which human beings act, through evoking in them certain wishes, desires and dreams'. This is happening all the time in our global world, with the powers-that-be and electronic media spinning a confounding magic that has had a 'lethal impact on democracy' (ibid., p. 23). The challenge is to escape this web and construct a new one, and the question this chapter – indeed the book – asks is whether arts-based research methods lend themselves to this task. This is not a straightforward process, however, and some of the pitfalls are interrogated here as it is asked whether this just results in the 'reproduction of the same knowledge with a different literary twist' (Mazzei and Jackson 2009, p. 2).

The section 'Hearing silences' includes discussion of the collaborative nature of storytelling and draws on an innovative storytelling project, *OurStory Scotland*, in order to consider the need to hear voices which have long been silenced and attempts, in so doing, to strengthen marginalised communities. One of the dilemmas here involves the notion that, as well as keeping people together, stories can also keep them apart (Frank 2010, p. 2). The notion that voice can ever be 'authentic' is also raised, and this continues to be an issue in the section 'Crafting stories', which as well as looking at the way crafts might be used to facilitate storytelling, considers the extent to which the resultant work 'speaks for itself'. Continuing this theme of representation, 'Capturing stories' considers how we might pin down ephemeral experience and narratives that are non-linear and tangled. There is a *range* of different voices that might be acknowledged through various methods of storytelling, including dreamlike voices and humorous voices, stuttering voices and nonsensical voices. In the section 'Changing the story' the need is stressed not just to listen for alternative voices, but to hear alternative stories. There is potential for these to challenge the status quo and to offer alternative and exciting visions of life. However, it can be surprisingly difficult to change the script.

Hearing silences

> My mum found out I was gay, by accident. Total and utter accident. Yep. And decided to use it against me, had control over me for four months of my life. I wasn't allowed to go anywhere. I wasn't allowed to see anyone. I wasn't allowed to do anything. But behind her back I was seeing my current partner who I've been with for over two years now. And I snuck off down to Glasgow one weekend ... and I had to tell her. And she told me she was going to tell my father and my father was going to take me back [to live with him in a remote area] ... I was really, really scared because I didn't want to go home and I didn't want to go back to her house either. So my partner said to me, 'phone your father. Talk to him'. So after twenty minutes of me babbling down the phone and of him asking, 'What is wrong with you?' I told him, 'I'm gay'. And he goes, 'Yeah, I know!' [audience laughs]
>
> (Video 1)

This is the story of one of the participants in *OurStory Scotland*, a large-scale storytelling project that uses a wide range of storytelling methods, including visual and performative approaches. The aim of *OurStory Scotland* was to research, record and represent the history and experiences of Scotland's LGBT (lesbian, gay, bi-sexual and transgender) community 'through their own words' (Valentine 2008, para. 13). It culminated in a ceilidh, a traditional Gaelic social gathering revolving around music and dancing, that included displays of the art work that had been created through the project and performances by storytellers in a 'magical combination of music, dance and stories' (ibid., para. 63). The project's title endeavours to highlight the collective resistance to the power of dominant classifications to define, those which 'name you as "other", implying a whole discourse and predefined narratives' (ibid., para. 11). The project uses stories to 'revise people's sense of self, and … situate people in groups' (Frank 2012, p. 33).

Storytelling is by its nature a collaborative enterprise. There is a sense of companionship in storytelling (Benjamin 1969/2006, p. 372) because of the necessary involvement of an audience. It is the relationship between the teller or re-teller and audience that shapes the stories told. Ken Plummer (1995, pp. 20–21) refers to the 'joint actions' of the storyteller and the 'coaxer' in constructing stories. The coaxer brings the teller 'to the edge of telling a story they might never have told before, and [encourages] them to tell it in a certain way'. This is one possible role of the researcher/facilitator in collaborative arts-based research, although there are certainly other possibilities, as the examples in this chapter testify. Arts-based methods of creating stories, including quite literally sewing them together, draw attention to the ways that stories are constructed artefacts – albeit always constructed in relationship to lived realities – rather than 'authentic' truths. They are always built on shifting ground, but although this should be acknowledged throughout the research process, it need not be seen as problematic. Error is accommodated within literature and storytelling, unlike the language of science which continuously endeavours to eliminate error (Winterson 1996, p. 166).

Dialogical narrative analysis is a way of understanding stories that builds on Bakhtin's (1984) notions of dialogue (Frank 2012, p. 33). It involves looking at how stories are co-constructed through turn-taking, adding, embellishing and polishing. Stories are thus understood as 'artful representations of lives'. Some of the factors that influence the success of the 'artfulness' of the storyteller include:

> the resources to tell particular kinds of stories, affinities with those who will listen to and understand such stories, vulnerabilities including not being able to tell an adequate story, and contests, including which version of a story trumps which other versions.
>
> (ibid., p. 34)

It is particularly important in research for social justice to consider why one story is told and not another, given that narratives are never neutral but rather depend on the positionalities – that plethora of intersecting factors – of not just the teller, but also the re-teller and the audience (Osler and Zhu 2011, p. 228). Voices and stories cannot be extracted from social and cultural locations or from interlocking oppressions (Maguire 2001, p. 62).

OurStory Scotland can be seen as helping to create group identities and boundaries. However, interestingly, audiences were often welcomed from outside the local communities where stories were collected, and they also comprised people outside of the LGBT community. The ceilidh, for instance, was made open to anyone who wanted to attend and was advertised in the local press. This, James Valentine (2008, para. 52) stresses, would have been 'unthinkable' at the start of the project, before group identities were strengthened and participants' confidence grew. One element of the project involved a community event to which participants were invited both from the locality and outside it. Fifty 'episodic' stories that had been collected in that particular community were made available to participants, and each chose one episode to read to the group as well as declaring their reasons for selecting it. It was found that participants tended to choose stories from 'across the conventional borders that can divide the LGBT community' rather than those closest to their own experiences. The narrative research process might thus be seen as an unintended exercise in community building, 'developing a sense of solidarity around a shared history and narrative heritage' (ibid., para. 25). This exercise also emphasises the performative nature of storytelling (see Langellier and Peterson 2004). Knowledge is not stored in storytelling but rather it is 'enacted, reconfigured, tested, and engaged by imaginative summonings and interpretive replays of past events in the light of present situations and struggles' (Conquergood 1993, p. 337). The 'narratives of narratives' (Valentine 2008, para. 27) in *OurStory Scotland* enables this reconfiguring. Even if the stories stay structurally the same, the re-telling by others will involve their particular tone of voice or intonation, in fact their very embodiment, thus conveying new meanings to a new audience in an occasion which offers a possibility for 'felt emotion, memory, desire, and understanding' to come together (Denzin 2003, p. 13).

The dialogical nature of storytelling means that, in line with Freirean pedagogy, it can introduce participants to 'critical insights that slice through entrenched taken-for-granted attitudes about everyday reality'. In the process of reflection we 'redefine ourselves, reposition ourselves in relation to reality' (Ledwith and Springett 2010, p. 110). Mary Jo Dudley (2003, p. 304), who carried out a participatory video project with Colombian domestic workers in order to explore their stories and challenge stereotypes, found one of the benefits of the research process was the provision of a forum 'to listen and learn from the experience of other group members, thus reinforcing the collective knowledge of the group'. The research also highlighted the extensive knowledge that participants *already* had, despite their lack of formal education. This sharing of stories can also be useful in helping people understand that 'their individual sufferings have social causes' (Mies 1983, p. 128).

One of the visual storytelling components of *OurStory Scotland* involved participants making papier mâché masks (Figures 3.1 and 3.2) in order to represent ways in which they have felt forced to present themselves. Many of the participants expressed 'ambiguity, duality or multiplicity' in the very look of their masks

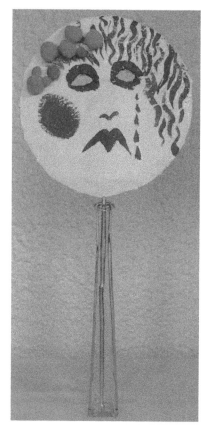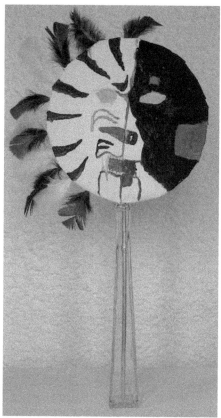

Figure 3.1 Mask of Criz (*OurStory*
      Scotland mask workshop)

Figure 3.2 Mask of Anne (*OurStory*
      Scotland mask workshop)

Source: Reproduced with the kind permission of *OurStory Scotland*.

(Valentine 2008, para. 48). A number of the participants chose to perform their stories through their masks and found that these visual artefacts aided their storytelling (Video 2). Some elected to hide behind them, others not. The masks, together with the performed stories, recall Frank's (2012, p. 33) discussion of dialogical analysis whereby it is understood that 'any one voice comprises multiple perspectives'. The perspectives that are offered up during a particular storied account necessarily reflect the occasion, the audience and the extent of the encouragement offered. Stories cannot be seen as 'the simple unfolding of some inner truth' (Plummer 1995, p. 34) but rather something tellers are brought to say in a particular way, at a particular time and place. The recognition that a single voice cannot represent a single truth has tended to be addressed by pluralising rather than universalising voice and offering a multiplicity of accounts, as in the case of *OurStory Scotland*. However, Lisa Mazzei and Alicia Youngblood Jackson (2009, pp. 1–2) point out that this approach of 'more is better' still assumes a 'present, stable, authentic' voice. Again, this is not a significant 'problem' if it is faced up to and acknowledged that however innovative, inclusive or progressive its methodological approach, research needs to avoid explicitly or implicitly claiming access to 'the truth'.

Another aspect of the *OurStory Scotland* project involved gathering stories from a range of participants and scripting them into dramatic monologues (Valentine 2008, para. 28). The monologues included scenes from different decades of the twentieth century, with older participants being interviewed about their lives. One man, Monte, in his eighties, was interviewed about life in the 1930s–1950s. A phrase from his story, 'keep quiet', was reiterated throughout the monologues, and Valentine delights in the 'delicious irony' of the 'public declaration of invocations to keep quiet' (ibid., para. 28). Monte watched the performance of the monologues and felt that his story was captured well, and no doubt the story also resonated with the audience to a greater or lesser extent. However, there is a further irony here, given that 'the voices that are given a hearing' in research have been 'censored and disciplined' even before the research questions are asked (Mazzei 2009, p. 46). Even such innovative methods as scripting participants' exact words into performance texts 'fails to consider how these exact words have been shaped through the research process' (Mazzei and Jackson 2009, p. 2). The resultant accounts therefore risk silencing those stories that do not fit with the aims of the research, not to mention those altogether less desirable voices. Communities themselves are not necessarily stable and authentic. Kwon (2004, p. 7), for instance, dismisses the idea of community as a 'coherent and unified social formation'. Rather it can serve 'exclusionary and authoritarian purposes in the very name of the opposite'. If a community chooses to present a particular face, even in terms of worthwhile social causes, one outcome is that 'silent' voices are ignored. They are not easy to make sense of and they transgress 'the domesticated voice that we are accustomed to hearing, knowing, and naming' (Mazzei 2009, p. 46).

Crafting stories

Storytelling is by no means an exclusively female activity, but Warner (1995, pp. 21–22) delights in looking at women's historical roles as storytellers, spinning 'old wives' tales' as they went about their routine, repetitive work.

> No one could say that the stories were useless
> for as the tongue clacked
> five or forty fingers stitched
> corn was grated from the husk
> patchwork was pieced
> or the darning was done …

> (Liz Lochead 2003, p. 79.
> Reproduced with kind permission from Birlinn Ltd.)

Although the feminist movement has insisted that women's talk 'is not mere gossip folklore' (DeVault 1999, p. 2), the storyteller remains, it is claimed, 'more exposed and vulnerable than the scientist in pursuit of covering laws and grand theory' (Conquergood 1993, p. 337). No wonder, then, 'that the epistemological power of narrative performance is denied by disparaging the "anecdotal"'. Darlene Clover's (2005; 2007; 2011) work evokes the world of Warner's tattlers as she employs craft-based methods in her work in adult education. Crafts *have* tended to be a largely female domain, with activities such as knitting circles 'referred to as gossiping circles, trivial and domestic' (Clover 2005, p. 633). Yet women across the globe have long used the arts as ways of telling stories, asking questions or creating knowledges. An example of this is the aperillas, or storied pieces of cloth, created in Chile under the Pinochet regime and smuggled out to inform the outside world of the atrocities being committed (Clover 2011, p. 13). Clover (2005; 2007) has also used the practice of quilting in her own work and has explored ways in which this can be used as 'politically active aesthetic practice' (Clover 2005, p. 634). It is a means of collecting data as well as a vehicle of dissemination and education. Completed quilts have been displayed at local art shows, international academic conferences and a large traditional quilt show. One of the important starting points for this practice is that it is a 'comfortable' craft with which women are often familiar (ibid.).

One quilting project involved young women and social workers at a family centre addressing the question, 'What does sexual exploitation mean to you?' (Clover 2007). This saw sixteen squares completed and stitched into a quilt with a deep fuchsia pink background. Clover describes the juxtaposition of the soft fabric, the security and comfort of the quilt, 'the familiarity, and the intimations of domesticity', with the stark world of sexual exploitation (ibid., p. 91). Images on the squares include a red splotch on a black background that symbolised the participant's pain and a recumbent pregnant woman with her legs open and vagina exposed (ibid., p. 90). A second quilting project, *Crying the Blues*, was carried out by a group of older women in response to the impact of the government's cuts to healthcare services in Canada, and the increasing privatisation of these services. Thirty-two squares produced by different groups of older people across Vancouver Island were sewn together by the project facilitator to form a 'creative tapestry of story, image, symbol, metaphor and experience'. Some of the squares are symbolic: a pair of scissors to indicate cuts; an 'H' with a line through it which Clover (2005, p. 634) points out represents the closure of hospitals but might also mean 'do not enter', alluding to the rise in infections within hospitals which might partly be attributed to the cuts in cleaning and support staff. Other squares are more pictorial, one illustrating a centenarian woman being denied homecare.

These projects have resonance with Suzanne Lacy's *The Crystal Quilt*, a 'tableau vivant' that took place between 1985 and 1987, and has more recently been screened at London's Tate Modern (Video 3). This collaborative public art work also had the aim of promoting dialogue with and listening to older women who are often rendered invisible in Western society. The original performance took place on Mother's Day. Women sat down at meticulously arranged tables, and as they sat down they unfolded red and yellow tablecloths, rested their arms symmetrically on the tablecloths, held hands and began to have conversations based on questions that older women had raised during the course of the project. These were not about 'memories', as much research with older people tends to dwell on, but very much focused on the present and future: older women as activists. Every few minutes a sound would signal that they should move the positions of their hands. Viewed from above (by three thousand spectators) this scene became a kaleidoscopic living quilt; the movement of hands represented stitches changing. The audience could not hear the conversations, but they were played a pre-recorded conversation based on reflections of seventy-five older women.

My own experimenting with arts-based research methods arose from a community art group that I ran for several years with socially and economically disadvantaged mothers and grandmothers of young children at a Sure Start programme in the UK. The arts group involved us working on a range of arts and craft activities, from découpage to jewellery making. Some of these activities I suggested, others were instigated by members of the group. The group proved more popular than I had ever envisaged, and attracted a particularly 'hard-to-reach' population. This included a wide age range of women who, otherwise, would not have had cause to meet, given that the local community was considerably under-resourced in terms of venues and social opportunities. Group members enjoyed being creative and learning new skills, but what took me by surprise was the remarkable ease with which story after story was told as we busied ourselves with painting flowers on glass vases or stencilling lettering onto greetings cards. Tales were often intimate and bawdy, or related hardship and tragedy, and we frequently laughed and cried together. Over time it gave me a depth of insight into the community that I cannot imagine having gleaned from any other means, and paved the way for the research project that I developed based upon these experiences. Yet this also proved a responsibility. I had not entered this arena intending to carry out research, and although running the art group was not officially an ethnography, it was akin to one. And there is a real threat of feminist ethnography masking 'a deeper, more exploitative form of exploitation' because of its dependence on 'human relationship, engagement, and attachment ... The lives, loves and tragedies that fieldwork informants share with a researcher are ultimately data, grist for the ethnographic mill' (Stacey 1988, pp. 22–23). The soothing, repetitive nature of crafting, the gentle creative buzz, enables a sharing of stories that might otherwise remain untold, and this can be risky.

Lisa Kay (2013) has also found that crafting lends itself to becoming a research tool, and has experimented with the use of beadwork to facilitate storytelling. This developed from her own 'life changing' personal experience of attending a beading workshop and creating her first piece, *Transformations*, from beads and found objects (Figure 3.3). She subsequently went on to use the technique in her role as an art therapist, and then later as a qualitative researcher and 'a/r/tographer'. In this latter role Kay devised a research project to look at the role of art education in alternative schools with 'at risk' students. This comprised a number of creative elements, including observations that were worked into poems. The project also

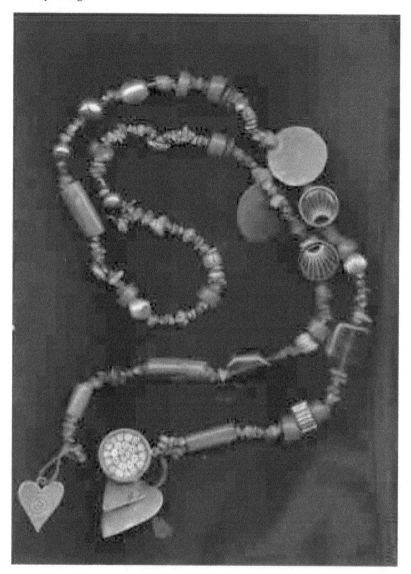

Figure 3.3 Lisa Kay's *Transformations*

Source: Kay 2013. Reproduced under the terms of the Creative Commons Attribution Non-Commercial License.

required that Kay interview art teachers. Initially dissatisfied with the interview process, feeling that something was 'missing' and wanting to find a more collaborative, dialogic approach, Kay returned to art making.

She provided her interview participants with a delicious assortment of beads: 'Long, short, glass, wooden, multi-colored, molded, striped, dotted, carved, cloisonné'. Participants were encouraged to choose beads that represented their values and experiences, and to string these together whilst they talked. So stories were spun from beads and a piece of string. And as with my experience of running the art group, Kay found that this talk flowed as participants engaged with both the creative process and their imaginations. A black onyx became a 'puzzle piece' that represented young people finding their place in the word. Silver tubular beads were 'dumbbells' representing strength. This visual storytelling process enabled 'artistic thinking in addition to verbal thinking' and participants were able to communicate 'tactilely and metaphorically' (Kay 2013, pp. 8–9).

Kay claims this process was 'empowering', arguably a grand and somewhat unsubstantiated claim. However, there is little doubt that the process was an enjoyable one for participants who were 'like kids in a candy shop' when presented with the beads. It also opened a space for rich dialogue, which Kay was able to capture through her field notes and subsequently script into a short play. The bead collages that resulted from the process acted as 'visual transcripts', adding to the project's 'constellation' of evidence (Kay 2013, p. 11). Whether this evidence is sufficient in terms of social research practice is questionable, however, and this is a stumbling block for much arts-based research, and qualitative research more generally. This issue of analysis and the extent to which stories – and the visual art work and performances discussed in Chapters 4 and 5 – can be expected to stand alone without being sufficiently theorised needs consideration. St. Pierre (2009, p. 227) is unequivocal in her assertion that rigorous analysis should not be neglected. She is dismissive of research stories that are intended to 'speak for themselves' and that suggest participants' voices are 'sacrosanct'.

There are certainly problems attached to claiming that voice is 'authentic'. However, at the same time, too much heavy-handed analysis and weighty explanation stifles some of the magic of story:

> Every morning brings us news of the globe, and yet we are poor in noteworthy stories. This is because no event any longer comes to us without being shot through with explanation. In other words, by now almost nothing that happens benefits storytelling; almost everything benefits information. Actually it is half the art of storytelling to keep a story free from explanation as one reproduces it.
>
> (Benjamin 1969/2006, pp. 365–366)

Derrida describes the contradiction inherent in the etymology of analysis: ana– referring to births, causes, a return to origins; –lysis a dissolving, a breaking down, a resolution. It is 'as if analysis were the bearer of extreme death and the last word … [yet also] turned toward birth' (Derrida, cited in MacLure 2009, p. 101). In this sense analysis can be understood as being regulated by the stricture of the double-bind: 'Pull on one thread and you tighten the other' (MacLure 2009, p. 101). This paradoxical image is one that would appeal to that trickster figure encountered in the previous chapter; the trickster that 'suggests our situation when we give up mastery but keep on searching for fidelity, knowing all the while we will be hoodwinked' (Haraway 1991, p. 199). MacLure (2009, p. 98) describes the qualities of voice that are typically lost through the process of analysis and representation. These are those 'double-dealing, mischief-making qualities' that would appeal to any trickster: 'jokes, lies, feints, detours, contradictions, exaggerations and misfires, laughter, gasps, tears, sneers and silences'. Arts-based methods do offer possibilities of capturing these elusive, confounding moments, if we are able to '[let] go of the literal rather than documenting it' (Rasberry 2002, p. 116).

Capturing stories

And at first light …
the stories dissolved in the whorl of the ear
but they
hung themselves upside down
in the sleeping heads of the children
till they flew again
into the storyteller's night.

(Liz Lochead 2003, p. 79.
Reproduced with kind permission from Birlinn Ltd.)

The stories that were told at the Sure Start art group were never captured in any form of documentation, although no doubt many of them will continue to be retold, subtly changing on each occasion. My memories of that time are momentarily revived by the smell of burnt toast or coming across a stall selling greetings cards at a craft fair; then a jumble of images and feelings washes over me, that would be nigh on impossible to pin down in words on a page. As Law (2004, p. 2) posits, conventional research methods do not take into account that 'much of the world is vague, diffuse or unspecific, slippery, emotional, ephemeral, elusive or indistinct, changes like a kaleidoscope, or doesn't really have much of a pattern at all'.

Kip Jones (2006a, p. 190) has arguably succeeded in pinning down some of the ephemeral elements of storytelling, through the use of performative methods when presenting the story of his interviewee Polly. When she was eight years old, Polly's father returned from the Second World War and it was at that point her parents decided to divorce. In Polly's description of the night that her mother left the family home, Jones notes the confused order of events – the telling of the way her mother 'walked out' comes before that of an earlier conversation during which Polly had been asked to choose which of her parents to live with – and the way that 'expressive passion overshadows chronological time'. Jones likens Polly's attempt to verbalise her experience to how one might endeavour to express a dream, 'clutching at details to make it more real' (2006a, p. 190). As MacLure (2009, p. 98; italics in the original) stresses, 'Voice always evades capture. Something is *always* lost in translation'. In Chekhov's short story 'The Kiss', the painfully shy, diffident officer Ryabovitch experiences his first kiss which has a ravishing effect on his life. He also makes the discovery – quite painful to him – about the gap that lies between thinking and telling.

> He began describing very minutely the incident of the kiss, and a moment later relapsed into silence ... In the course of that moment he had told everything, and it surprised him dreadfully to find how short a time it took him to tell it.
>
> (Chekhov 1999, p. 66)

Janet Malcolm (2004, p. 44) reflects on Ryabovitch's dilemma: 'The gossamer images that sit in one's head have to be transformed into some more durable material – that of artful narration – if they are not to dissolve into nothing when they hit the chilly outer air.' Indeed, Jones' answer to the dilemma of capturing Polly's story certainly lies in 'artful narration'. He presents the work as a short film, *I Can Remember the Night* (Video 4). This is voiced over by three actors of different ages – a young girl, middle-aged woman and older woman – representing different stages of Polly's life. The actors are all from the same northern English working-class family. The result is moving and powerful; it captures the dreamlike aspect of Polly's narrative, and her unsuccessful attempts to pin down her vivid but just-out-of-reach memories have been partially resolved by the comprising of grainy black-and-white domestic photographs – interior and exterior shots – from the 1950s and 1960s (Figures 3.4 and 3.5). The work can be accessed via You Tube and at the time of writing has had over a thousand views, an unequivocally large audience for an account of social research. This genre of work might satisfy

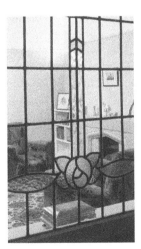 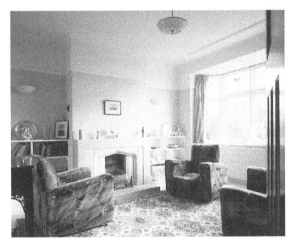

Figures 3.4 and 3.5 Stills from Kip Jones' *I Can Remember the Night:* John Lennon's home with his Aunt Mimi until 1963, restored by The National Trust, with furnishings and interior decoration similar to the way the rooms looked when Lennon lived there

Source: Photos courtesy of the National Trust, 251 Menlove Avenue, Liverpool.

Back's (2007, p. 7) call for a more 'imaginative engagement' with social life and novel ways of communicating this to the public.

For research that aims to promote social justice, engaging a wide audience is key. The turning of 'tales of suffering, loss, pain, and victory into evocative performances' has the ability 'to move audiences to reflective, critical action, and not just emotional catharsis' (Denzin 1997, p. 95). In a report published by the Joseph Rowntree Foundation (Castell and Thompson 2007, p. 42), it is suggested that in order to develop greater public support for anti-poverty policies, it is necessary to have 'real examples' in the form of 'narratives and stories that enter popular myth'. By telling our stories in an accessible way, whether through readable books, theatre, film or on television, we can make a significant contribution to public knowledge and public debate (Behar 2003, p. 34). If social research is to realise its emancipatory promise, 'what we are going to need are strong, personal, heartfelt voices, the voices of love, trust, faith and the gift' (Behar 2003, p. 37). There are, however, limits to this empathy and these are explored in Chapter 5.

The focus on creating innovative stories does run the risk of textual strategies losing 'empirical bodies' and displacing important questions, such as 'who is speaking to/for/with whom, for what reasons and with what resources?' (Lather 2007, p. 44). There is a need for more interactive social relations in order not just that new voices are heard, but that voices are 'hearing one another fruitfully'. Lather (2007, p. 42) reflects on *Troubling the Angels* (Lather and Smithies 1997), the book that came out of an experimental feminist ethnographic project about how women living with HIV/AIDS make sense of their lives. The book plays with textual practices, splitting the text so that the women's words are presented in large type at the top of the page, and the researchers' accounts in smaller type below. National statistics, drawings and poetry add further facets to an account which aimed to 'say more and other about something as absurd and complicated as dying in the prime of life' (Lather 2007, p. 41). One means by which this was achieved was through the process of inviting members of the group to 'check' the book's authorial voice, this itself adding 'a layering of further data into the text'. Drawing on Gallagher (2000), Lather (2007, p. 42) reflects:

> Inviting the women in our study to see themselves being studied, 'looking-at-being-looked-at-ness' becomes both 'a way of seeing and a way of representing' that is 'troubled, exalting, particular and communal,' where not only researcher and researched but also readers are 'left open for scrutiny' in what we think we know.

Whilst Jones has elsewhere advocated 'cross-pollination' in terms of working together (cited in Leavy 2009, p. 18), and *I Can Remember the Night* was certainly collaborative in the sense that it involved a team of people, it would have been interesting to know the extent of Polly's involvement in the finished piece. Like more conventional research, the end 'product' of arts-based research is often taken out of the hands of those providing the data. Given Jones' skilful treatment of the story, this is not necessarily a flaw, but again is worth acknowledging.

Anne Davis Basting's (2001) creative storytelling project, *Time Slips*, similarly involved project facilitators having a role in putting stories together, but through a process that consciously aimed to respect participants' input. They avoided the temptation to impose a linear narrative, but rather left language 'free to carry emotional, rather than literal, meaning' (Basting 2001, p. 83). This research overtly set out to hear the voices of marginalised people, in this instance those experiencing Alzheimer's disease and related dementia (ADRD). Basting organised several months' worth of weekly storytelling workshops with people with symptoms consistent with middle-stage Alzheimer's, all of whom required 24-hour care. The resultant stories, almost a hundred in all, were worked into a play, and incorporated within an art installation and a website to strengthen public awareness of the capabilities of people with dementia.

Basting (2001, p. 79) notes that people with ADRD lose the ability to comprehend chronological time systems. This is thus a much exaggerated version of Polly's difficulty in telling her story chronologically. Gradually, people experiencing ADRD begin not only to forget details, they also start to forget concepts: 'One does not just forget where one put the keys. One cannot comprehend the *meaning* of a key.' Given the care that is required for people with ADRD, they also provide an extreme example of a relational 'self', one that is formed through interaction with others. However, as she points out, we all understand ourselves through our relationships with other people and institutions.

The aim of the research was not to pressure participants to remember their pasts, but to focus on who they are now, 'complete with missing words, repeated sounds, and hazy memories', and to collaboratively fashion new stories by employing the communication skills that they had retained and the ways that they currently functioned. For instance, one storyteller's language was limited to the sounds 'Babababababa' but this was able to be incorporated into nearly all the stories (Basting 2001, pp. 80–81). This focus on the present time recalls Lacy's *The Crystal Quilt* project discussed above, where attention was on older people's present lives. There is power in the present, particularly in terms of making positive change. The now is the *only* place where change can happen (Tolle 2001).

Each week, the group's facilitator would encourage the group to choose an image from a selection, on which the story would be based. The story would be constructed by participants' answers to a series of questions posed by the facilitator. The retelling of the story, as with Jones' *I Can Remember the Night*, required some artistry from the project's facilitators. Basting (2001, p. 81) describes the 'certain theatrical flair' that was needed to interpret 'a random list of sensical and nonsensical answers'. This process also involved facilitators having to let go of the literal and forsake linear narrative. Basting admits that it was overwhelmingly difficult to resist the urge to tidy up the stories, to 'craft them ... to draw out and polish the rich metaphors and symbols that lay like geodes in the riverbed of the tales' (ibid., p. 89). It is this resistance, however, that lends the project its fascination: '[T]ruth is always deeper and richer than any description of it. To change lenses and face a fuller spectrum of that truth … requires daring' (Starhawk 1987, p. 26).

> *That's a Big Body...*
> (In response to an image of an elephant and a little girl)
>
> We are deep in the heart of Austin, Texas.
> Grandfather the elephant lives at the zoo and does tricks in the circus.
> But he's not allowed to sing there.
> One day, while walking down the street, he meets Amy, a 10-year-old girl.
> Now, most people would run away when they meet an elephant on the
>   street, but Amy has no fear.
> They become friends.
> One day, Grandfather takes his car and drives from the zoo to the church,
>   where Amy is at a wedding.
> He waits for her outside, because he's too big for the church.
> If he went in, he'd break it down.
> While Grandfather waits, he hears 'Abide with Me' coming from the
>   church. *(Group sings 'Abide with Me.')*
> He likes it because he's not allowed to sing at the circus.
> Amy comes out to meet him and feeds Grandfather corn and hay and grass,
>   because grass is good.
> Grandfather has floppy ears.
> He's a very good person, he's comfortable and happy.
> Amy falls asleep on Grandfather, and he waits for her to wake, then gets
>   back in his car and drives back to the zoo.
>
> (Basting 2001, p. 84.
> Reproduced with kind permission of the author.)

The surreal feel to this work – the way that it captures participants' loosening grasp on 'reality', and stitches together such incongruent flashes of memory with compassion and humour – comes some way to achieving MacLure's (2009, pp. 97–98) goal of 'voice research'. This would attend to:

> laughter, mimicry, mockery, silence, stuttering, tears, slyness, shyness, shouts, jokes, lies, irreverence, partiality, inconsistency, self-doubt, masks, false starts, false 'fronts' and faulty memories – not as impediments or lapses to be corrected, mastered, read 'through' or written off, but as perplexing resources for the achievement of a dissembling, 'authentic' voice.

Basting (2001, pp. 82–83) describes the collaborative storytelling in the project as an 'incantation'. During the process the usual rules of time and authority were suspended. This evokes the liminal festival of carnival, which is explored in Chapter 6 in relation to collaborative arts-based research. By taking 'time out of time' and putting reality on hold, an interlude is created 'where laughter, play and fantasy might reside' (Riggio 2004a, p. 15) and change is possible. In Basting's research, this would be a space to celebrate the various ways in which people with ADRD actually function rather than putting any pressure on them to remember their pasts.

Changing the story

The *Arabian Nights* comprises a large collection of folk and fairytales from myriad sources from across North Africa and Central, West and South Asia that were translated into French and English in early Enlightenment times. Although the tales have gone through countless changes over the centuries, the central premise remains the same. It is one where stories are literally life and death. The Sultan is enraged by the infidelity of his wife, and as revenge has vowed to marry a virgin every night and have her slain in the morning. As the supply of young women dwindles, Scheherazade, the Sultan's eldest daughter, volunteers herself. Bringing her younger sister with her, Scheherazade proceeds to tell her a bedtime story. The Sultan is captivated by the storytelling and night-by-night puts off her execution because he wants to hear more:

> The power of stories to forge destinies has never been so memorably and sharply put ... the blade of the executioner's sword lies on the storyteller's neck.
>
> (Warner 2011, p. 5)

Gargi Bhattacharyya's (1998) work draws on the 'error-filled, corrupt pleasures' of the *Arabian Nights*. Employing a Black feminist approach, and the innovative form of a series of stories, she draws attention to the 'complex mechanisms that are at work in shaping racial images and myths' (Solomos 1998, p. viii). These myths, Bhattacharyya (1998) would argue, have been constructed from countless years of societies telling and re-telling oppressive tales of sex and violence; hyper-sexualised or threatening Black bodies always requiring restraint.

> If the stories you believe define your range of possibility, then you have to change the story to something else. In the stories of great men work had no value and so people who worked were less than those who were employed or who had no need of a wage. In the old stories, being poor was a punishment for working and the wealth of those who did not need to work was a reward for their special talents and extra cleverness. The confinement and subjugation of women was determined by nature; and was therefore unquestionable and unavoidable. The formerly colonized and enslaved had limited capacities and, although this was sad, it was also the way of the world. These repeated stories crossed over and reinforced each other, until the lives of the rest of the world seemed to be tied down to nothing at all. The great men rode plots of achievements and adventure, while the rest of the world were stuck tight in their destinies of disrespect. Telling the story

the great men's way meant erasing the work and contribution of the rest of the world. Of course, when you rubbed out all the people underneath, it looked as if the great men could fly.

(Bhattacharyya 1998. Reproduced with permission from Taylor and Francis.)

Research for social justice requires alternative stories when the accepted versions are wounding and oppressing whole swathes of people. In this sense, lives really do depend on storytelling. Ruth Behar (2003, p. 15) discusses the 'flagrant colonial inequalities' that underpin ethnography and give privileged researchers the power to tell stories of the 'other'. The need to challenge this power remains crucial, but difficult given that '[e]ach attempt at renouncing the colonialist gesture that suppresses or erases subjects' voices seems to end up re-offending' (MacLure 2009, p. 102). We can only acknowledge our limitations whilst continuing to strive for positive change; to problematise aspects of our stories; to explore the political nature of everyday encounters. It is through this process that we 'move towards the critical consciousness necessary to demystify the dominant hegemony, revealing life with all the stark contradictions that we live by' (Ledwith and Springett 2010, p. 111).

Haaken and O'Neill (2014) raise some highly pertinent concerns in relation to the research carried out with asylum seekers using an approach which O'Neill has elsewhere termed 'ethno-mimesis' (see O'Neill et al. 2002). This storytelling project deals with tales laden with 'heavy political cargo' (Haaken and O'Neill 2014, p. 79) in an attempt to document women's feelings of well-being and safety. Participants comprised women from West Africa, South Asia and the Middle East who were at various points in the process of applying for asylum. The researchers approached asylum seeking 'as a daily process rather than a final decision granted by the border control agency'; they were all too aware that in their role as researchers they had the 'potential to collude in the persecutory apparatus of the state' and thus they consciously aimed to 'expose the illusions that elicit identification with state power' (ibid., p. 80).

The project required alternative stories to the frequently trotted out media presentations of asylum seekers as 'bogus', not least due to the fact that the state itself makes 'bogus claims of protecting citizens from dangerous border crossers' (Haaken and O'Neill 2014, p. 86). This aim was facilitated by arts-based methods that included a walking tour of the local area with participants following a map they had collectively produced. The map located meaningful sites; sites that had particularly positive or negative associations. Participants were provided with disposable cameras so that they could capture significant images on the walk. Photographs were subsequently analysed through a group process and displayed in an exhibition, and a video was made by one of the researchers to document the research process (Video 5). Whilst this process elicited rich stories, the very fact that the stories were so engaging caused Haaken and O'Neill concern. Were they relying on the 'most evocative and readily visible effects of immigration policies' (ibid., p. 83)? Were they in danger of reproducing the very representations they wanted to guard against? They give the example of a story told early on in their project by a woman whose baby had died when she gave birth at home:

> It was a heart-wrenching story that dramatized the fate of so many women migrants across the globe … This story of a mother's loss – a woman seeking sanctuary and being turned away in her most vulnerable state – vivified the moral failures of the state.
>
> (ibid.)

The researchers suspected that, through stories such as this one, the women were aiming to meet 'a perceived expectancy for morally unambiguous stories'. Given that the asylum seekers' position is frequently feminised and associated with 'desperate states of dependency, vulnerability and need' the story comfortably meets the 'officially authorised scripts for female suffering'; the researchers, however, were keen to open space 'for a more complex refugee subjectivity' (ibid., p. 87).

Participants in research alter their stories according to what they believe is expected or what they think the interviewer 'can bear to hear' (Grenz 2005, p. 2096). They also have in mind how their stories might be interpreted and how they will be perceived by the wider public. This dilemma echoes my own experiences during the Sure Start research project, most notably when participants made short films based on their day-to-day lives and their interactions with the Sure Start initiative. Two of the women chose a 'redemption' narrative, whereby they described how Sure Start had saved them from a life of drugs and destitution. These made for powerful tales which were met with an enthusiastic reception from their audience. However, it was reading between the lines of these stories that I found much more interesting, and I discuss the disjuncture between the films' images and the narrative in Chapter 6. Although it was clear that the women had moved forward in their lives, their relationships with the Sure Start initiative remained tense and they frequently (when not on film) complained about feeling judged by the staff. Moreover, the initiative had not, as far as I had observed, had any role in the women choosing to cease (or, more accurately, to reduce) their drug use. These tales chime with what Lather (2007, p. 8) describes the 'too-easy-to-tell story of salvation', a temptation for researchers and participants.

'Behind Closed Doors' (Eisenhauer 2012, pp. 7–10) is a digital story that aims to address issues of the representation of people with psychiatric disabilities and the stigma and silencing they face (Figures 3.6 and 3.7). The form of video is an apt one, given that living with a mental 'illness' requires constant 'screening', from stigmatised depictions on television and film through to routine invasive screening by medical staff. Popular culture and medical discourses have not been short of stories to tell about those experiencing mental health conditions. The resultant research of 'Behind Closed Doors' is thus not solely about sharing information, but about a kind of defiant speech, a form of talking back, when dominant discourses and the resulting stigmatisation teach us to be silent. What is particularly noteworthy in the work is the *discomfort* that the research created

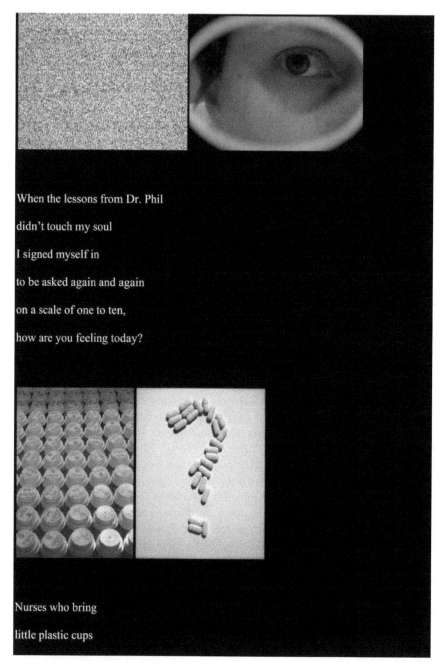

When the lessons from Dr. Phil

didn't touch my soul

I signed myself in

to be asked again and again

on a scale of one to ten,

how are you feeling today?

Nurses who bring

little plastic cups

Figures 3.6 Caption on the next page

filled with calm or happiness or sleep,

take their coffee on the cool side

but again and again I remember

there is a lock on that door

that I am not allowed

close enough to see.

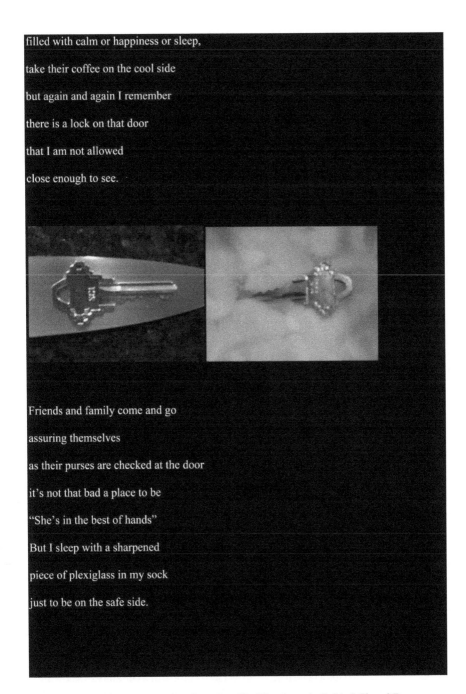

Friends and family come and go

assuring themselves

as their purses are checked at the door

it's not that bad a place to be

"She's in the best of hands"

But I sleep with a sharpened

piece of plexiglass in my sock

just to be on the safe side.

Figures 3.6 and 3.7 Images taken from Jennifer Eisenhauer's *Behind Closed Doors* (2012)

Source: Reproduced with permission from Taylor and Francis.

through this confrontation. Within an ableist culture, 'the silence surrounding mental illness may be more comfortable than the unlearning involved through the intervention of such an artistic practice' (ibid.). Eisenhauer draws on Kumisharo (2002) in order to think about the pedagogical implications of digital storytelling if we are to 'understand learning not as "affirming what we already know," but rather as "something that disrupts our commonsense view of the world"' (ibid., p. 12). Thus are 'common sense' understandings revealed as cultural myths.

Conclusion

The chapter begins with an opening scene from Carter's *Nights at the Circus* where the journalist, Walser, is first confronted by the larger than life character of Fevvers. Fevvers' and Walser's relationship develops through the book as Fevvers maintains her charade of being a winged creature, 'Hatched out of a bloody great egg'. Like Scheherazade before her, Fevvers knows that 'to come to the end of her story is to face her own kind of death ... So she has to cast a spell with her voice' (Finney 1998, para. 11). It is through this opening scene that we are 'plunged into the narration of a very unusual narrator whose peculiar combination of Cockney English and classical erudition suggests her status as half human and half mythical'. This can be seen to mirror the nature of narrative itself (ibid., para. 6). Carter's own discussion of the text has included her desire to invite readers 'to take one further step into the fictionality of the narrative, instead of coming out of it and looking at it as though it were an artefact' (Haffenden 1985, p. 91). Elsewhere she has talked about the need to 'travel along the thread of the narrative like high wire artists' (Carter 1993, p. 2).

The chapter has looked at a range of examples of arts-based storytelling in research. The resultant tales invite immersion into their worlds. They are constructions, just as accounts produced by more conventional methods are, but they arguably offer something extra, some temptation to listen. They therefore provide an opportunity to reach out and engage with an audience in order to raise awareness of marginalised groups and challenge stereotypes. Stories 'offer a way of putting questions, of testing the structure as well as guaranteeing its safety, of thinking up alternatives as well as living daily reality in an examined way' (Warner 1995, p. 411). Yet there is still a potential for stories to exclude. They may try too hard to please their audience, or conversely to repel their audience by being too confrontational. MacLure's (2009, p. 98) solution to this conundrum is to propose a 'poetics of insufficiency' rather than a 'poetics of sincerity'; the latter 'produces innocent voices that speak a familiar script of redemption or triumph, in tones that lack idiom and surprise'; a poetics of insufficiency, on the other hand, 'would recognise the irreparably split nature of the self and the broken voices in which it speaks'. There is perhaps a need to give up 'on the promise of a certainty of knowing' (Mazzei 2009, p. 59). Arts-based research lends itself to this submitting to the mystery of the world. Bradley Pearson, a character in Iris Murdoch's novel *The Black Prince*, muses: 'Only stories and magic really endure. How tiny one's area of understanding is art teaches one perhaps better than philosophy' (1999, p. 13).

4   Image and metaphor

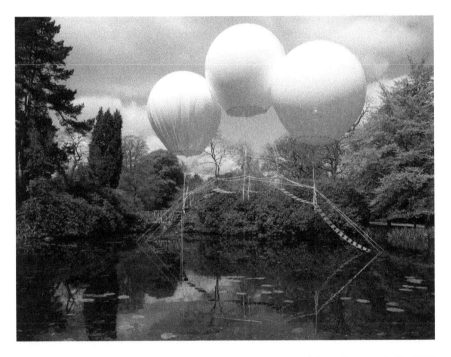

Figure 4.1 Olivier Grossetête's *Pont de Singe*. Planks of wood (cedar), ropes, balls, TPU
Urethane, Helium, PVC pipe, screw hooks and anchors, variable dimensions
(for biennal : 20m/5.6m/13m), Tatton Park Biennial, Manchester, 2012

French artist Olivier Grossetête's mesmerising *Pont de Singe* is a fantasy bridge, a
fairytale bridge, a folly of a structure that would not be out of place in one of
Calvino's surreal *Invisible Cities*. Suspended over a lily pond by three helium
balloons, in the Japanese garden of a historic estate in northwest England, this
'monkey bridge' would undoubtedly appeal to the trickster – that figure who has
been appearing intermittently through the book in relation to the contradictions and
dilemmas that arts-based research poses for social justice. It absurdly subverts the
purpose of a bridge (indeed the very notion of gravity) whilst cunningly enticing

its viewers to cross it. Grossetête's bridge evokes some of the ideas discussed in this chapter, including Elliott Eisner's contemplations on the 'product' of arts-based research. He notes that the conclusions that can be drawn from this form of inquiry tend to be metaphorical, and 'more ethereal, global, impressionistic' than the 'more literally oriented', purposeful answers that conventional research provides (Eisner 2008b, pp. 22–23). These metaphors should 'generate new dimensions of understanding. They should augment – or trouble – our capacity for explanation' (Siegesmund and Cahnmann-Taylor 2008, p. 241).

Whilst the *Pont de Singe* does not fulfil its function as a bridge (although Grossetête does note that the structure is able to support one person's weight), as an aesthetic work of art it has a very real purpose in terms of engaging viewers' thought and rallying an emotional response. In the way that it simultaneously lures and perplexes the viewer, the bridge mirrors the tension between accessibility and elusiveness in the arts in terms of what art, imagination and creativity can offer to social practitioners. Art 'readily strikes a chord, more easily than words' (Chamberlayne and Smith 2009, p. 5). It encourages participation and engages an audience. Yet at the same time, 'exploring deeper meanings of art ... can be elusive and challenging' (ibid.).

Grossetête's aim with *Pont de Singe* was to provide a meditation on turning daydreams into reality, 'to make alive the poetry and dreams within our everyday life' (Dezeen 2012). As discussed in Chapter 1, there is a political purpose for doing just this. David Darts (2004, p. 315), for instance, outlines the role of the arts (he is writing in the context of art education) in 'the uncovering of ideological struggles within the realm of the everyday'. He cites the Russian critic Viktor Shklovsky (1988), who claimed that it was only through art that we could begin to become aware of that we had become 'habituated' to. The recent visual turn in the social sciences and humanities draws on this premise. The task of the visual cultural theorist might be understood as being to 'overcome the veil of familiarity and self-evidence that surrounds the experience of seeing, and to turn it into a problem for analysis, a mystery to be unravelled' (Mitchell 2002, p. 166).

Visual studies thus tend to emphasise the politically and socially constructed nature of reality, whether the focus is on photographs, art works, film or the everyday world of signs and objects (Emmison et al. 2012, for example, encourage researchers to move beyond two-dimensional images and think about the vast array of visual data available, from everyday objects and domestic spaces and beyond to wider social spaces such as parks and city centres). Enabled by the postmodern turn, this is a major shift away from understanding the image as a direct representation of reality. Photographs and film were traditionally used as objective evidence in anthropology, or for illustrative purposes in sociology. John Berger's (1972) *Ways of Seeing*, based on a television programme of the same name (Video 6), was groundbreaking in terms of its explanations of fine art paintings, the impact of photography and the contextual nature of visual images, which can no longer be understood as 'a technically effected window on the world' (Chaplin 1994, p. 199). The process of producing an image might tell us more about the image maker than his or her subject, 'given that the particular visual cultures they are bound up with will shape their choice of subject, how they locate the subject within the frame and what they choose to leave out' (Warren 2005, p. 864, cited in Packard 2008, p. 72). In terms of interpretation, images can also be seen as 'something like a Rorschach ink blot in which people of different cultures spin out their respective worlds of meaning' (Harper 2002, p. 22).

Visual sociologist Elizabeth Chaplin (2004, pp. 35–36) describes having kept a visual diary for fifteen years, capturing the everyday routine that 'much of our lives consist of' but that is rarely documented in the way that momentous events are. Not only is this attention to the quotidian important for social scientists, but the art of taking and viewing photographs leads 'straight to the heart of social science theory'. Tension certainly resides 'between what a photo shows and what a photo means' (Chaplin 2005, para. 1.1). Chaplin's visual diary has taken various poetic and unconventional forms over the years and has on occasion been exhibited in a gallery setting. She has explored a number of theoretical ideas through this work. At one stage, when Chaplin was closely involved with artists producing non-figurative work, she began taking abstract photographs of different walls. Each day, a close-up image of a particular wall was accompanied by an image which provided a contextualising view. This spoke to Chaplin's preoccupation not just with aesthetics, but with the way that context is crucial in terms of interpreting an image or text. Background transforms a foreground object 'from an aesthetic composition to a social situation' (Chaplin 2004, p. 38).

It was not long before Chaplin reintroduced traces of herself into the photographs, 'a shadow, a footprint, an actual reflection (in water or a mirror) or an actual hand or foot'. This enabled her to address pressing feminist methodological concerns, such as the position of the researcher in the research process and the question of voyeurism. Visual social scientists have certainly been prominent in exploring these ideas and also in considering ways in which gathering visual data can help to mitigate the traditional power imbalance between researcher and researched (see Pink 2007, pp. 109–112). There is much potential for participation in this approach to research, as well as an opportunity to provide a critique of the status quo. Over time, visual social science has moved 'from a focus on the specific, which hid and muted the critiques of the system, to exposing social problems and injustices by inclusion of context and research subject "in the picture"' (van Son 2000, p. 217).

Some of the techniques developed in this context, such as photo elicitation, are discussed in this chapter. There are substantial links here with the previous chapter in terms of the examples of visual storytelling that were introduced and the dilemmas these raised concerning notions of 'giving voice'. Simons and McCormack (2007, p. 296), examining the use of arts-based methods in evaluation research, note the benefit of enabling participants to portray their experience through various art forms:

> [T]hey often reveal insights that they cannot articulate in words. For people or groups who are less articulate, who learn in different ways, or who have different cultural backgrounds, it can be a most useful means of engaging them … and offering them a voice.

Whilst this chapter advocates this active involvement of participants in research that employs image and metaphor, it also extends the argument that such emancipatory claims are not straightforward. The chapter also aims to move beyond a literal understanding of the visual. Sarah Pink (2007, p. 21), despite being a leading figure in visual ethnography and methodology, understands that there is an 'undue stress' on the visual in terms of visual research methods. They are *not* purely visual. In fact, there is something of a paradox here, not least in one of Mitchell's (2002, p. 170) eight counter-theses to visual culture that involves a 'meditation on blindness, the invisible, the unseen, the unseeable, and the overlooked'. A quite literal demonstration of this supposition is provided through Peter Wheeler's (2012, pp. 285–286) account of negotiating the qualitative research process as a blind researcher. He effectively argues that 'observations and interpretations are possible without sight', and that by not making causal links between sight and vision, openings emerge for a more diverse research community. Les Back (2007, p. 8) would agree that a reliance on the visual is not sufficient for an ethical research practice in a diverse society. Social researchers who employ what Back terms a 'democracy of the senses' are 'likely to notice more and ask different questions of our world'. It is here that the imagination can play its part. Angela Carter, several of whose plays were broadcast on radio, claimed that the radio was 'the most visual of mediums because you cannot see it' (cited in Clapp 2012, p. 18). This summation is echoed in the reactions of an audience member to a choreographed performance of research findings produced by Carl Bagley and Mary Beth Cancienne. Whilst this involved an innovative communication through dance, the spectator felt that had she been able to read the written text rather than watch the performance, she would have been more able 'to imagine the participants' voices and meanings'. It was the choreographers who had had the creative role in the process of telling the research stories, and thus, admit Bagley and Cancienne (2002, p. 17) it 'hindered rather than facilitated the use of her imagination'.

The first section in this chapter, 'Challenging conventions', discusses two projects that utilised participatory photography with marginalised groups and some of the dilemmas and successes that arose through this practice. These examples, like many in the chapter, involve elements of storytelling. However, discussion also incorporates the extent to which images and metaphors produced through research might speak for themselves. Shaun McNiff (1998, p. 44), for instance, is troubled by 'the assumption that visual, kinetic, or auditory communications must always be translated into verbal language to be understood'. He describes an 'artistic knowing' as a contrast to intellectual understanding (ibid., p. 17). The use of metaphor in visual research is also important in 'Negotiating ethics'. This section of the chapter tackles some of the complex ethical debates that arise through this way of working. Although this has relevance, to a greater or less extent, to all of the methods discussed in this book, visual methods in particular draw our attention to pressing issues of consent and the extent to which subjects are identifiable. The section 'Poetic licence' introduces various ways that poetry might be used as method and, in doing so, continues to think about the notion of metaphor in research. It also considers the emotional aspect of communicating research findings, the flow of feeling that poetry might create and conversely the stickiness it produces when attempting to represent the lives of others.

Eisner (2001, p. 136) raises this emotional dimension of the arts in a discussion concerning some of the parallels between art and qualitative research. He argues that emotional qualities of art are inseparable from aesthetics. Through aesthetic engagement with viewers, artists are able to convey the 'sense' of situations; make them 'palpable'. Aesthetic, emotional and affective dimensions of arts-based inquiry are woven through the chapter, but the section 'Affective aesthetics' provides more direct focus on these particular facets. Again, there is an ethical dimension to this discussion; emotions are very much implicated with issues of justice and injustice (Ahmed 2004, p. 195). To suggest that they are not would support the universalist ethics of Kantian and post Kantian traditions whereby emotion is divorced from reason. There are different ways of approaching aesthetics, and certain perspectives have more resonance than others in research for social justice. Grant Kester (2004, p. 112), for instance, outlines a 'dialogical aesthetic' which does not require universal standards of objectivity. Achieved through actual dialogue, it is 'based on the generation of a local consensual knowledge that is only provisionally binding and that is grounded instead at the level of collective interaction'. Richard Siegsmund and Melisa Cahnmann-Taylor (2008, p. 240) draw on Hannah Arendt's (1968) work on aesthetics as a philosophy of creating communities of caring. This is far from a 'conventional definition of a philosophy of beauty', but art can be seen as 'a vehicle that propels research'. This is also the case here, with the added caveat that the research aims to promote social justice.

Challenging conventions

There is a range of participatory visual methods that offer possibilities for collaborative research for social justice. Douglas Harper (2002, p. 13) provides a useful definition of photo elicitation and its development in visual anthropology and visual sociology. This method involves employing a visual image – most usually a photograph – in a research interview in order to elicit not *more* information, but a *different kind* of information. This works (or does not work) 'for rather mysterious reasons' (Harper 2002, p. 22), but these reasons are likely related to the fact that 'images evoke deeper elements of human consciousness than do words'. Harper's enthusiasm for the method is due to its collaborative, dialogical nature; the way knowledge is constructed through human interactions. This aspect has also appealed to critical researchers. The Freirean method of liberating education involves facilitated dialogue about a familiar, everyday scene that is captured through a drawing, photograph or other art form: 'the issue becomes decontextualised, or coded, and can be seen more critically as a result' (Ledwith and Springett 2010, p. 18). 'Draw-and-tell' (e.g. Driessnack 2006) is another collaborative visual method, most often used with young children who are asked to draw particular experiences and describe them in conversation with the researcher.

Photovoice is a method committed to social transformation, and it has become increasingly popular with feminist researchers, particularly in the health field (e.g. Wang 1999) and community development (Walton et al. 2012). It employs photo elicitation methods as well as group discussion 'as a form of knowledge generation, connection, and consciousness raising' (Ponic and Jategaonkar 2012, p. 190). Yet power relations are not so easily mitigated. They, along with 'conventions of spectatorship', remain 'embedded in the institutional production and reproduction of research artifacts' (Haaken and O'Neill 2014, p. 82). Such techniques need to be used with care and reflection. Josh Packard (2008), in respect of his visual research with homeless people in Tennessee, provides a very thoughtful and moving account of some of the dilemmas he encountered. The aim of his project was to generate knowledge that could ultimately improve the living conditions of its participants. Aware of the loss of dignity that being homeless can engender, Packard set out to ensure that some of the power relations in the research would be alleviated by enabling participants to fully take part in a process that would increase their self-esteem. Participatory visual methods offered that promise. Packard managed to recruit twenty-four homeless participants to his study through a process of snowball sampling. He carefully explained the purpose of the project and handed each participant a disposable camera with the brief to take pictures of 'things, people and places that are important to you in your daily life' (ibid., p. 66). In return for their role in the project, participants received five dollars and a set of prints. Packard received eleven of the cameras back with around 250 useable images and, through a laborious process of tracking down their locations, he managed to conduct interviews with ten of the photographers.

The interviews involved looking through the sets of pictures and encouraging the photographers to speak about them. One of the unforeseen issues regarding this process was the lack of skill that participants had in terms of handling the disposable cameras. Although Packard (2008, p. 70) had been assured by participants that they were competent in photography, the resultant pictures told a different story. For instance, every single one had been taken in the 'landscape' as opposed to 'portrait' position and the flash had very rarely been used which meant that the photos that had been taken at night were rendered indecipherable. Packard describes in poignant detail his follow-up interview with 'Ralph', whose finger had partially obscured the lens on every photograph he had taken (Figures 4.2 and 4.3). Packard had been anxious about the interview, rightly predicting that Ralph would be embarrassed by this rudimentary error. Moreover, the composition of the photographs meant that it was unclear what their focus was, and Ralph struggled to explain what the images he had taken represented:

> [T]he link here between knowledge and power could not be made clearer. [Ralph's] lack of knowledge about how to use an item, which he understood was clearly intended to be an uncomplicated version of a more sophisticated object that many people use on a daily basis, greatly affected his ability to tell his own story. Not only did his technical incompetence directly obscure the

information in the image, but his feelings of shame and embarrassment inhibited him from communicating his perspective.

(ibid., p. 71)

Packard notes that lack of expertise in photography was demonstrated by all the men to some degree, and this has 'profound methodological and substantive consequences' (2008, p. 74). The methodological implications include not being able to fully communicate their stories, thus 'giving voice to the voiceless' became an impossible mission because of the 'extreme marginality' of participants. Substantively, the men's lack of familiarity with the process reflects their marginal position in society, as did the 'awkward' shots taken at a distance. Image after image depicted 'empty' landscapes and the lack of close-up shots echoes the distance from society that the homeless men experience. Packard draws on Bourdieu and his assertion that the conventions employed in photography indicate what method and style is 'common to a whole group'. The *lack* of conventions in Packard's participants' photographs certainly mirrors their exclusion from the dominant group.

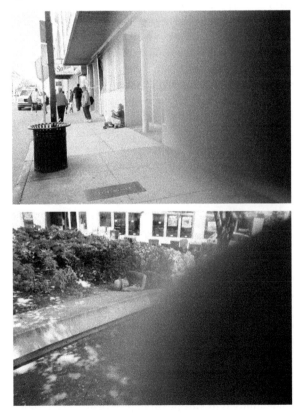

Figures 4.2 and 4.3 Examples of photographs taken by Josh Packard's participants

Source: Packard 2008.

Whilst Packard concludes that the men in his project did not have the resources to act as co-collaborators in the research process given that 'they had neither the knowledge nor power to fulfill this role', his sensitive and evocative write-up of the project, together with a series of photographs, does raise readers' awareness of the very marginalised existence of homeless people. This was an incredibly 'hard to reach' community, and differed considerably from Quaylan Allen's (2012) participants in his participatory photography project. These were comprised of Black middle-class teenage boys at a school in the United States. This is not to suggest that it was a non-worthwhile community on which to focus. Black boys and men, as Allen makes clear, are frequently 'sensationalised within a hegemonic racist discourse' and represented as 'deviant, irresponsible, sexually superior but lazy and uneducable' (ibid., p. 452). The project offered an opportunity to tell a different story, one outside of this racist and gendered discourse, but in attempting to do so it also raised its own set of dilemmas.

Once again, the 'conventions' displayed among the participants in terms of method and style can be seen as being applicable to the whole group. They also play to stereotypical images of the group. For instance, Allen found that the boys he wanted to recruit to the project did not engage in the pilot study when he handed disposable cameras out. These cheap and cheerful cameras were 'not 'cool' enough' to 'affirm their masculine performances', performances that emphasised 'the aesthetics of materiality, the acquisition of expensive clothes, shoes, and nice cars as a symbolic representation of being successful' (2012, p. 454). The young men had the resources to be able to handle the equipment; digital photography has become a cultural norm amongst young people with cameras on mobile phones being widely used, and digital platforms such as facebook and instagram providing opportunities to disseminate images. However, they did initially lack confidence in terms of their role in the project. Allen argues that it was his role as researcher, and his commitment to social justice, to 'empower' participants:

> The method is not empowering in and of itself, but finds its power in the negotiation between the moral commitment of the researcher and the agency of the participant.

> (ibid., p. 452)

In this case, Allen, as a Black man himself, was able to convince his participants of the social and political need to hear the Black male voice, as well as to show a 'deep interest in their wellbeing'. Whilst the researcher's role is undoubtedly key in terms of negotiating power relations, his or her ability to *confer* power is questionable, as is the necessity of researchers and the researched sharing similar backgrounds. The project was regarded as successful in terms of producing knowledge that was able to be disseminated to the participants' teachers in order to give them more insight into the lives of young Black men. The participants were gratified and enthused by this possibility of being better understood. It did, however, prove difficult to move beyond stereotypical representations, despite the commitment of the researcher. Allen admits that 'the method doesn't ensure that Black male youth won't visually represent themselves in ways consistent with dominant discourse on Black masculine performance' and gives the example of how the participants 'sought to establish masculine coolness through heteronormative performances with female students', intent on flirting and identifying themselves as 'ladies' men' (ibid., p. 453). Perhaps then the most useful question for researchers remains why one story is told and not another (Mazzei and Jackson 2009, p. 4).

Negotiating ethics

Creative methodologies that use images produced by participants or researchers intensify the debates surrounding research ethics. So far in this book, although its prime objective is to offer suggestions for research practices that make positive contributions to people's lives, the various proposed ways of working have not been discussed in relation to any specific ethical models or frameworks. This is in part due to the lack of desire to be prescriptive, but also because each project has its own set of concerns to work through. In general though, the projects that are discussed throughout the book can be seen to follow an 'ethics of care' approach in which 'ethical decisions are made on the basis of care, compassion and a desire to act in ways that benefit the individual or group who are the focus of research' (Wiles et al. 2008, 2.2). The way that these decisions are made tends to depend on context and dialogue with participants, a situated ethics rather than a universal ethics. An ethical research practice, one that aims to unmask 'broader systems of power, privilege and oppression', needs to respect the participant's autonomy and acknowledge the notion of self-determination and choice (Ponic and Jategaonkar 2012, pp. 191–192). It requires 'extended, ongoing and reflexive dialogue between researchers and participants', not just a one-off decision by a research ethics committee.

That said, any research that is carried out in collaboration with an academic institution or the health service *will* also require approval from the relevant bodies. Reliance on established ethical frameworks is important and necessary. Andrew Clark (2013, p. 77), whilst being very much in favour of a situated approach to ethics, draws attention to the danger inherent in rejecting universal ethics as 'overly protectionist' or 'unfit for specific contexts'. This could lead to the 'permissive use of unprincipled or unscrupulous practices conducted in the name of situated ethical practice'. There is therefore a need to hold these very distinct approaches to research ethics in tension with each other. However, although institutional frameworks potentially offer protection to participants and researchers, they frequently lack sufficient relevance to visual researchers (Clark 2013, p. 68). Rose Wiles et al. (2008), in their review of key ethical issues in research employing film, photographs or video images (created either by researchers or participants), acknowledge that most ethical protocols are not specific enough to include directives on visual methods. They also discuss the anxiety expressed by visual researchers concerned that the demands of ethics committees will limit the possibilities of visual research and render data meaningless (Wiles et al. 2008, 2.4). As a means of addressing some of these dilemmas, Clark (2013, p. 77) emphasises the need to 'recognise participants as active, ethically reflexive agents who negotiate the ethical conundrums of everyday life'.

This position is one that Pamela Ponic and Natasha Jategaonkar (2012) take in their photovoice project, *Shedding Light on the Barriers to Housing for Women Fleeing Violent Relationships* in four diverse Canadian communities. They also made sure that rigorous ethics and safety protocols were developed and put in place prior to undertaking any research, and that training was provided for researchers and participants. There was a heightened need in this project to ensure genuinely informed consent, safety and confidentiality, because all of the participants had experienced domestic abuse. Coupled with the fact that participants lived in small communities and were thus more readily identifiable, this meant that their role in the research could place them at risk (ibid., p. 190). The process employed in developing the protocol is one that could be readily adapted to other situations. It was developed in negotiation with participants, recognising the need for them to have agency in and some control over this process. Drawing on Olav Eikeland's work (2006), Ponic and Jategaonkar discuss the notion of 'condescending ethics' that can be the result of more traditional research ethics processes (ibid., p. 191). These tend to position participants as 'other' – for example, by enforcing anonymity when groups who have been chronically silenced prefer to claim their experiences as their own. Clark (2013, p. 71) shares this concern over such potentially 'dehumanising' practice, which may include disguising faces through pixilation, an ironic approach to take in an experience that intends to be inclusive and emancipatory.

Ponic and Jategaonkar's research aimed to act as an exercise to raise awareness of the barriers to housing that women face after leaving violent relationships. Thus the (visual) findings were to be shared among policy makers, government workers, organisations and the general public. Clark (2013, p. 73) points out that because visual images lend themselves so keenly to being shared with an audience (and this might be in a variety of contexts, including dissemination on the internet), then questions over who has 'the "right" to use, display and reuse' this data are paramount. There is perhaps an unspoken assumption that the researcher is better able to re-present the images than the original makers, to tell their story more comprehensively. Thus, as well as working through 'heightened threats' of anonymity and confidentiality (Ponic and Jategaonkar 2012, p. 192), there is a need to be able to 'critically justify ... the need for the production as well as the display of visual material' (Clark 2013, p. 74). Ponic and Jategaonkar's solution to some of these issues was to use the concept of photo as metaphor. Training in this approach was provided by an artist/activist, and the outcome was a series of highly creative and powerful staged photographs that protected participants' identity yet heightened the 'ability for action and advocacy' (2012, p. 200) through the affective dimension of sharing such deeply felt experiences in an aesthetic and poetic way. One photograph depicts a child's pair of jeans, carefully arranged on a bed, but dirty and tattered. It evokes the photographer's pain and shame of not being able to provide adequate clothing for her child. Another image shows the tread of a man's heavy boot on a female hand, its fingers stretched out towards a key just out of reach.

Images and metaphor often possess an affective power to 'move an audience or viewer or evoke certain reactions and that in turn prompt further response and actions' (Clark 2013, p. 74). Arts-based methods are able to 'move us at an emotional and sensual level' because of their independence of rational and linguistic systems (Gunaratnam 2009, p. 26). This is both an ethical and epistemological issue. Images can be interpreted in a variety of ways and may even manipulate by evoking guilt in viewers (Clark 2013, p. 74). An alternative, but equally troubling, possibility is that art might indoctrinate rather than emancipate, 'lull into quietude'; confrontational art may even alienate viewers (Barone 2008, p. 40–41). If art does draw its audience in, it is also a possibility that an image might go on to 'haunt' its viewer (Clark 2013, p. 74) and this is something that we should thus be attuned to in terms of anticipating the ways that research findings may be interpreted.

Emotional and affective responses to arts-based research can also be understood as assisting in producing knowledge.[1] It is through these moving reactions and bodily responses that information can be created and conveyed. Emotions have usually been considered 'potentially or actually subversive of knowledge'. It is thus reason rather than emotion that 'has been regarded as the indispensable faculty for acquiring knowledge' (Jaggar 1997, p. 188). One of the significant contributions of feminist and anti-racist methodology is in its contestation of the opposition between rational thought and emotion. Not only has emotion been 'projected onto the bodies of others', who are then pathologised as a result (Ahmed 2004, p. 170), such a projection also 'works to conceal the emotional and embodied aspects of thought and reason'. It is certainly one of the strengths of arts-based inquiry that it draws attention to the 'emotionally wrenching ways in which we attain knowledge of others and ourselves' (Behar 2008, p. 63).

Poetic licence

Arts-based researchers not only acknowledge emotion, they 'seek to magnify the intensity' of affective experience in contrast to more traditional researchers who 'seek to "cool down" data via their presentation in research reports' (Furman et al. 2007, p. 302). In this book I have included excerpts of poetry, such as Barbara Marsh's 'Wall' in Chapter 1, in the hope that this can speak to the reader in ways that prose is unable to. Poetry has also proved a popular means for researchers to present their data in ways that condense research findings. Patricia Leavy (2009, pp. 66–67) offers a useful overview of different approaches to using poetry in research. She discusses the differences between narrative and lyric poetry; the first is more concerned with storytelling than the second which tends to focus on 'moments of emotion'. Narrative approaches encompass interpretative poetry, investigative poetry and ethnographic poetics, all ways of disseminating research data that provide researchers with 'a new way to account for merging the "voice" of their participants with their own insights' (Leavy 2009, p. 66). Susan Finley's *Dream Child* (2000) is a good example of such 'poetic dialogue'. It tells the story of a young woman encountered through an arts-based research project with homeless youths in New Orleans. Here is an excerpt:

> I think Ferret was the only squatter I ever knew who was clean.
> His name was Ferret, and he had a Ferret named 'Human.'
>
> I hope he'll take me back. At least think about it, but I hope he'll
> take me back.
>
> Bright morning light sneaks through slatted boards nailed loosely
> over glassless window frames forming streaked patterns on
> stained dark floors. Stretches feline into sun's warmth,
> pulls light blankets tight
> protects against
> damp morning chill
> breezes
> in with the sun's rays.
> She sleeps in a too large sweater, stretched
> by knees tucked against chest in the
> cold, lonely night.

(Finley 2000, pp. 433–434. Reproduced with
permission from Sage Publications.)

These are techniques that employ 'images, slices of conversation, repetition, and affect' and thus 'present both a literal and metaphorical way of seeing the world' (Lyons 2008, p. 80). Eisner (1991, p. 227, cited in Janesick 1998, p. 36) argues the case for 'metaphoric precision' in describing the social world: 'for making public the ineffable, nothing is more precise than the artistic use of language'. Laurel Richardson describes metaphor as 'the backbone of social science writing' (1990 p. 18), whereas James Clifford (1986, p. 100) views ethnographic accounts as allegorical in the sense that the stories they tell have 'the propensity to generate another story in the mind of its reader (or hearer)'. Allegory is an art form closely related to metaphor; a 'reading between the literal lines' (Law 2004, p. 88). If this invitation to recognise allegory in ethnography is accepted, light is shone on the fact that 'rich' and 'convincing' research accounts are 'extended metaphors, patterns of association that point to coherent (theoretical, esthetic, moral) additional meanings' (Clifford 1986, p. 100). Whilst in Western culture it is literal representation that predominates, 'direct representation is never direct. It is mediated … The appearance of direct representation is the effect of a process of artful deletion'. In that sense, representation is *'allegory that denies its character as allegory'* (Law 2004, pp. 88–89; italics in the original). This is a controlling ploy:

The powerful (try to) insist that their statements are literal representations of a single reality. 'It really is that way', they tell us. 'There is no alternative.' But those on the receiving end of such homilies learn to read them allegorically. Cynicism, scepticism, the detection of hidden interests, a sense of the ideological, these are the techniques used by subordinates to read through the words of the powerful to the concealed realities that have produced them.

(ibid., p. 89)

Employing poetry in ethnographic texts can thus be seen as drawing attention to the ways that 'new realities' are crafted. Kristina Lyons (2008) describes the method as providing a set of lenses so that an idea or concept can be experienced affectively, cognitively and imaginatively. It is particularly useful for exploring relationships. Deborah Austin's (1996) interpretative poem *Kaleidoscope: The Same and Different* explores her interactions with her fellow doctoral student, Mari. The very title conjures up the idea of multiple reflections, flashes of beauty and symmetry. Austin is an African American woman, whereas Mari grew up in Central Africa. The poem attends to the two women's spoken conversations as well as to Austin's 'thoughts, memories, and judgments', which she acknowledges contributed to the ways that their relationship played out. She aims to capture the mesmerising musicality of Mari's voice 'which sounded like the hush of many waters', whilst exploring Black women's identity. This is a short extract from the lengthy poem:

We do look alike
>   high cheekbones under taut brown skin
>   cheekbones that my family
>>   claimed
>>   were a sign that we had Indian blood
>>   in the days when nobody
>>>   wanted to be African
But I am the daughter of slaves
>   as some Africans
>>   so quickly remind us
Still, she says
>   as she looks at the pictures
of me
>   pasted all over my kitchen refrigerator
while I cook barbecued chicken, collard greens,
>>   macaroni and cheese
>   butternut squash, homemade biscuits, and iced tea
>   the kind of dinner
>   my grandmother would make
>>   I hope she does not consider me vain
>>   And I tell her that
>>   the pictures

story part of my life
in a purple silk dress
sitting in the grass
at Boston's Arnold Arboretum
smiling at Loretta
who says that anyone
can take good pictures
of someone they love
You look like
A true African woman

(Austin 1996, p. 208. Reproduced with
permission of AltaMira Press.)

Adrie Kusserow (2008, pp. 74–75) began writing ethnographic poetry in response to feeling stifled by the 'scientific', 'stale' anthropological writing that she had been working on. She delighted in the way that she was able to retrieve '[a]rt and emotions, thick wild description, the whole messy terrain of the unsaid'. This felt 'like a bloodletting', she says: 'All of the colour, moods, feelings and nuances I'd wanted to gush for some time, came out easily'. Carl Leggo (2008, p. 170) also describes poetry in this embodied way, as being 'rooted in everyday experiences, connected integrally to the flow of blood in our bodies, expressed constantly in the rhythms of our speech'. This notion of movement is crucial to Sara Ahmed's (2004, pp. 10–12) thesis on emotion and the ways that emotions can be understood as shaping cultural politics. Although 'emotion' comes from the Latin emovere – 'to move, to move out' – emotions are also about attachments and connections. Movement connects us to one another yet it may also 'affect different others differently'. This is because emotions in their 'very intensity' involve miscommunication, 'such that even when we feel we have the same feeling, we don't necessarily have the same relationship to the feeling'. In exploring the ways that emotional responses are implicit in reproducing 'intractable and enduring' power relations, Ahmed (2004, p. 12) raises the question of why social transformation is 'so difficult to achieve'. The 'stickiness' that she describes is also a useful metaphor for poetic research methods and the difficulty of mitigating the power imbalances in research relationships.

Through the process of presenting sensitive data via poetry, researchers are obliged to see the researched as co-participants rather than subjects. However, researchers are not going to 'automatically become more empathic towards participants' (Furman et al. 2007, p. 302). Writing strategies are 'moral decisions' (Richardson 1990, p. 38, cited in Rath 2012, para. 5) but, as Kakali Bhattacharya (2008, p. 86) concludes in her account of being a research poet, the only voice she can truly 'claim' is her own, 're-presented through/ with/ against the contested voices of the participants, which inevitably leads to messy spaces of knowing and being known'.

Enabling participants to write their own poetry can be a partial solution to this stickiness, although, as discussed above, the accounts produced may not necessarily 'move' the stories of the researched out of the constraints of hegemonic norms. This method belongs to the category of *vox participare* (Prendergast 2009, p. xxii), participant-voiced poems, and offers a powerful, often therapeutic means of working. During the course of the research I carried out with mothers of young children at a Sure Start programme in northwest England, the women produced poems that still 'haunt' me and on re-reading have the power to evoke their voices and their being. We collaborated with a local poet who held a weekly creative writing class, and over time participants (mothers and grandmothers of young children attending the Sure Start programme) began to build skills and confidence in their writing. One participant described the group as the 'highlight' of her week. Another spoke about becoming 'creative with my feelings. I love writing poems as it helps me to deal with certain issues that's happened in my life.' The group culminated in participants having the resources to compose and perform poems about their lives and experiences of motherhood.

Pretty normal day

There's cat litter on
the kitchen floor
a roller skate next to
a fingerprinted door,
crumpled cornflake crumbs
in the video player,
and a suspect yellow
puddle right near
the potty.

I can't put used cups
in the sink because
it's full of last night's
dishes, unwashed.
She's screaming in my arms,
he's scaling the stereo,
chasing the cat
up high and down low.

He bumps his head
on the reading lamp
and we all sit there, my hair
curly and damp
from our tears.
                    (Sure Start mother)

Affective aesthetics

In a similar vein to research poets who work with the emotions raised during the research process, Moshoula Capous-Desyllas (2015) has produced an artistic account of the research she carried out with sex workers in Portland, USA. Participants in the study, after ethical and training issues had been addressed, took photographs of their 'lived experiences, needs, and aspirations' (ibid., p. 193). Photo elicitation and group dialogue sessions then followed in order to discuss images produced, and then the photographs went on to be displayed in various public locations over a two-year period. At the same time as this process was taking place, Capous-Desyllas – who describes herself as 'artist-activist-feminist-researcher' – produced her own visual art work, in the form of collage, as a way of '(re)imagining, (re)presenting, and critically reflecting' on her experiences (ibid. p. 195). The very process of creating a collage can be seen as a metaphor for unexpected alliances; 'connections that may otherwise have remained unconscious' (ibid.). The colours and images that Capous-Desyllas selected all had symbolic significance.

Figure 4.4 illustrates one of these collages, *Possibilities for an Outsider*, that encapsulates a number of important issues that Capous-Desyllas faced in carrying out the photovoice work. She also produced collages that represented later stages of the research process. This particular collage was worked directly onto a mount (or frame) rather than – as is usually the case – being framed after completion. This represents the researcher's feelings of unease and apprehension at the lengthy process still to come: the possibilities of collecting worthwhile data and the intensive interactions with participants, including sex industry workers, activists and social services providers. This way of working, of framing the work at the beginning of the process of making the collage, helped Capous-Dellyas to contain these anxieties and to acknowledge the early stages of the project as complete. This evokes my own experiences as an arts-based researcher. My research, as with the other projects described in the book, took a great deal of time and energy to work through, and extensive emotional labour in terms of forging and maintaining meaningful relationships. This is not always recognised in research accounts, so Capous-Desyllas' literal framing of this issue is valuable.

Capous-Desyllas chose a neutral grey background in order to represent the 'neutral' position she intended to take in the research as an outsider. She intended to react to situations without judgement or assumption, although she was simultaneously aware that personal biases would surface. The repeating diamond pattern reflects the faith that Capous-Desyllas initially had for the photovoice method: 'I thought that if I just followed the steps like a diligent researcher, what could possibly go wrong?' (2015, p. 197). However, one memorably negative experience happened when she and a colleague approached a group of exotic dancers outside a strip club and attempted to hand them flyers about the research project. They were met with a hostile response, the dancers swearing aggressively as they asked the researchers what they were doing at the venue. This left Capous-Desylla shaken and questioning her motives:

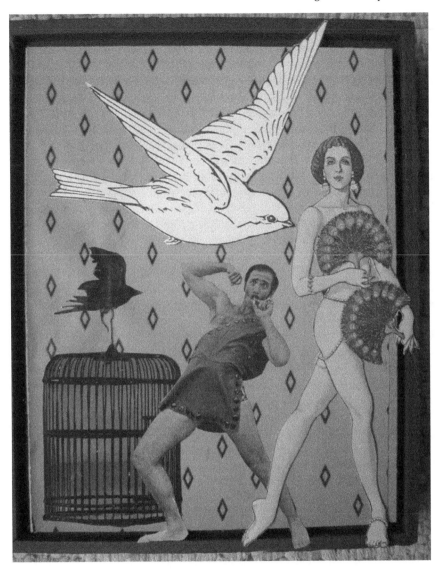

Figure 4.4 Moshoula Capous-Desyllas' *Possibilities for an Outsider*

Source: This image originally appeared in Capous-Desyllas (2015). Reproduced with permission from Taylor and Francis.

How could I (blindly) enter this space, shaped by socioeconomic status and race, and (naively) think that I would just be accepted? What did this reveal about my own privilege? How might the different color of our skin, our social and class privilege have played a role in how we were perceived, distrusted, and rejected?

(ibid., p. 198)

The white bird and the black birdcage in the collage represent opposing perspectives on sex work; sexual freedom and independence versus sexual slavery and victimhood. The caricature of the strong man and the connotations of power and control in this image evoke the concern that Capous-Desyllas had of perpetuating stereotypes through her research. (Given the examples discussed above, this is a very real worry.) It also suggests the awareness of the power she held as a researcher and the extent to which she could wield this to 'give voice' to the participants in the photovoice project. Capous-Desyllas sums up the project as making her feel uncomfortable about unequal power relations and the unanswerable questions surrounding this issue. Yet at the same time she remains immensely grateful for the opportunity to meet the sex workers and hear their stories: 'I cannot forget the power of this project' (ibid., p. 207).

Jennifer Lapum et al.'s (2012; 2014) arts-based research into the experiences of open-heart surgery patients did not employ a participatory methodology, but it did involve a highly collaborative process in its aesthetic and emotional approach to analysing and disseminating data (Lapum et al. 2012). The researchers included an evaluation of the impact of the arts-based dissemination, and this charts the embodied reactions of viewers (Lapum et al. 2014). The research culminated in an art installation incorporating poetry, photography and fabric in its labyrinthine design. This was displayed in two settings to an audience of patients and their families and healthcare professionals. Figure 4.5 shows the entrance to the work, which is 1,739 square feet in area and over 9 feet in height (Lapum et al. 2012, p. 100). Its title, *The 7,024th Patient*, comes from a quote from one of the thirty-two narrative interviews that were carried out with patients. Ninety-four journal entries were collected from participants. The interdisciplinary research team included: an arts-based researcher who was also a poet and a nurse; a multidisciplinary artist; a disability activist and arts-based researcher; a cardiovascular surgeon and professor; and a fashion academic with an interest in the body and design.

Free verse poetry was the leading method of dissemination because it was able to prioritise the words, phrases and ideas of participants, and this guided the content of the photography and the fabric art. Researchers listened carefully to the vocal register of participants and looked for metaphor and repetition in their speech. Imagination was a key aspect of this process as researchers attempted to 're-see' patients' experiences of open-heart surgery (2012, p. 104). These were experiences that had deeply affected participants and their stories were 'defined by introspection and personal transformation' (ibid., p. 101). The arts themselves have affective and transformative qualities and so researchers aimed to draw viewers into 'the emotional and embodied experience of an *other*, allowing them access to an internal experience' (Lapum et al. 2014, p. 12).

The installation takes the viewer on the journey of the patient, 'the rational as well as the bodily and messy aspects of human experience' (Lapum et al. 2012, p. 106). It begins at the point of leaving home to go to the hospital, then charts the preoperative procedures that take place, through to postoperative experiences and returning home then embarking on a changed life. The operating room is at

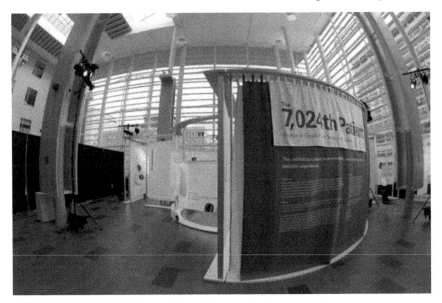

Figure 4.5 Jennifer Lapum et al.'s *The 7,024th Patient* art installation

Source: This photograph originally appeared in Lapum et al. (2014). Reproduced under the Creative Commons Attribution Open Access License Agreement.

the centre of the work and viewers have no choice but to pass through it on their route. This route is 'symbolic of patients' transition into the (iconic) center of the body (the heart), or deep within oneself' (ibid., p. 108). The structure of the poems aims to forge a physical connection between viewers and participants in the way that it follows the rhythm of participants' breath:

> I'm still, raw
> can't do what I want
> have to build up, feel
> like my chest was Ripped
> open
> just have to walk
> stop
> breathe
> step
> breathe
>
> (Lapum et al. 2014, p. 4. Reproduced under the Creative
> Commons Attribution Open Access License Agreement.)

Viewers certainly did respond to the installation in an affective, visceral way. The researchers recruited a focus group of men and women who had undergone open-heart surgery in the past (some were recent patients; others were fifteen years on in their recovery) to discuss their thoughts and feelings about the installation. Researchers also captured ad hoc responses of a number of visitors to the art work. Many of these were healthcare professionals. The responses centred on emotion, which can become 'the entry point to deeper insights into the lived reality of others' (Sharma et al. 2009, p. 1645).

For patients this was often due to the memories the art evoked (Lapum et al. 2014, pp. 4–7): 'I was getting these little flashbacks ... it reminded me of the exact time when I woke up because the clock was there, and the first things I felt'. Another expressed how the poetry brought back negative memories, 'because I mean, the whole operation was horrible ... the words are like, they're painful'. Others described physical sensations such as 'shivers' as they walked through the installation. One former patient described how 'I immediately feel emotion – bubble up in my throat', whereas another reported, 'It gets to the gut. It opens up what it is to be human.' Health professionals reported feelings of 'shared humanity' evoked by the work (ibid., pp. 8–10). It is easy, said one health professional, to lose sight of the fact that patients are 'alive with feelings and worries', but this poetic work acts as a forceful reminder.

One respondent, a former patient, acknowledged the resonance of the poetry, but was critical of the researchers' summaries that accompanied the work. These had been provided to help viewers make sense of the work, but the respondent felt that they interrupted his experience (Lapum et al. 2014, p. 5). However, he did admit that the analytic interpretations might prove useful for other viewers. The arts-based researcher can be seen as taking on the role of art critic (or literary critic in the case of poetry and story) in order to 'create and critique, challenge and explain' (Siegsmund and Cahnmann-Taylor 2008, p. 234). This is no easy task, and ascribing meaning to others' experiences often requires a cautious touch so as not to lose the 'magic' that the artistic work produces and so as not to privilege the researcher's (already privileged) position (Sharma et al. 2009, p. 1645). Both the artistic work and the accompanying explanations produced through arts-based inquiry need to promote conversation that enables us to 'see more deeply' (Siegsmund and Cahnmann Taylor 2008, p. 240). Certainly 'metaphoric novelty' is not sufficient for arts-based inquiry to be considered a success, even if it is aesthetically pleasing. Therefore aesthetic evaluation needs to be based on the success of its pedagogical functions (Leavy 2009, p. 17). The 'goodness' of poetry, for instance, revolves around its ability to open up 'a useful space that is shared between reader and poet' (Willis 2002, p. 9, cited in Furman et al. 2007, p. 303). Discussing dialogical art practices, Kester (Video 7) describes the collaborative experience itself, 'in all of its contradictory, politically compromised, rich, confused, haptic, discursive messiness', as an aesthetic experience. These are all generous understandings of aesthetics that take into account much more than how things look. Kester's fellow art critic, Bishop (2012, p. 19), however, is concerned by the perception that the social task of contemporary participatory art projects is 'more substantial, "real" and important than artistic experiences'. In terms of arts-based research then, the challenge lies in finding a balance between the closely related elements of the aesthetic success of the work and the ethical, affective and pedagogical outcomes.

Conclusion

Jo-Ann Archibald (2008, pp. 8–10), in her book on indigenous research, tells a story of the trickster character Coyote. This sort of transformer figure often employs 'humour, satire, self-mocking, and absurdity to carry out good lessons' (ibid., p. 5) and is a regular fixture of indigenous stories. In this story, Coyote learns a trick from Rabbit whereby he is able to make his eyes fly out and land on the branch of a tree. He happily shows off this new talent until a crow comes along and eats up his eyes. A sorrowful Coyote garners sympathy from the various animals he meets, and is donated a too-small eye from Mouse and a too-large one from Buffalo. He thus goes on his way with mis-matched eyes. Talfoya (1982, p. 24, cited in Archibald 2008, p. 10) views the story in terms of the holism that is important in indigenous cultures: to be whole and complete 'one must learn to switch back and forth between the eyes of not only Mouse and Buffalo, but … all the other animals of legend'. Archibald (2008, p. 12) uses the tale of Coyote and his uneven sight in order to consider the challenges of bringing together 'in harmony and balance' the tensions between the orality of indigenous culture and the literacy of academia; the discord between indigenous theory and research method. In terms of arts-based inquiry, the story could also represent the ways in which issues can be viewed from more than one position. What is seen depends on the angle of the viewing, and the desirability of seeing the world from different angles lends purpose to the task of 'artistically crafting' descriptions (Eisner 2008b, p. 22). These are descriptions that provide textures of lives rather than, as can be the case in sociological writing, 'flattened and glossed' accounts (Back 2007, p. 17).

It could also be argued that, like allegory, arts-based research 'extends the fields of visibility' (Law 2004, p. 90). Law posits that sometimes allegory 'also does something that is even more artful. This is because *it makes space for ambivalence and ambiguity*. In allegory, the realities made manifest do not necessarily have to fit together' (ibid., italics in the original). Again, the same could be said for arts-based research 'in its ambiguities, discontinuities and reversals' (Gunaratnam 2009, p. 25). The arts can be 'more open than linguistic representation to holding the threatening dynamic between "knowing" and "not knowing" that can involve denial, avoidance and detachment from difficult or painful realities' (ibid.). Perhaps, like Grossetête's bridge, floating unencumbered by weighty structure, art is able to 'open to us dimensions of the spirit and of the self that normally lie smothered under the weight of living' (Winterson 1996, p. 137).

Note

1   It should be noted that here, and in discussions in subsequent chapters, with Greco and Stenner (2008, p. 10) I use the terms 'affect' and 'emotion' interchangeably, although as these authors point out, many theorists, whether psychoanalytical or philosophical, might view this as problematic. However, insisting on a terminological distinction 'may actually obscure more than it clarifies at a conceptual level'.

5 Performance

Life is a cabaret.

(Sally Bowles, *Cabaret*. Words by Fred Ebb. Music by John Kander.
© Copyright 1966 Alley Music Corp, Trio Music Company – USA.
Reproduced by kind permission of Carlin Music Corporation, London
NW1 8BD. All Rights Reserved. International Copyright Secured.)

Give 'em the old razzle dazzle
Razzle dazzle 'em
Give 'em an act with lots of flash in it
And the reaction will be passionate
Give 'em the old hocus pocus
Bead and feather 'em
How can they see with sequins in their eyes?

(Billy Flynn, *Chicago*. 'Razzle Dazzle' by Fred Ebb
and John Kander. ©Warner/Chappell Music Ltd.)

If arts-based research methods have ineffable, 'magical' qualities, then nowhere are these more pronounced than in performance. There is something transformative that happens when everyday issues are performed on stage. Metaphorical sequins and greasepaint dress up the most humdrum of affairs, gilded by the hypnotic gleam of the spotlight. This chapter presents examples of how song and dance, performance poetry, performance art and art installations, drama and digital film can be employed in a collaborative research practice that seeks to further social justice. It thus aims to examine the extent to which 'truths' can be communicated through this razzle dazzle, and the potential of realising the utopian vision of live performance as providing 'a place where people come together, embodied and passionate, to share experiences of meaning making and imagination that can describe or capture fleeting intimations of a better world' (Dolan 2005, p. 2).

Amanda Kemp (1998, p. 116) describes how she uses performance 'both as a way of knowing and as a way of showing'. This is a useful way of thinking about arts-based collaborative social inquiry, with its methods that encompass understanding *and* representation (Denzin 2003, p. 33), even if representation is never as straightforward and unproblematic as we might like. Participants, researchers or facilitators are given the opportunity to explore their own lives and the lives of those around them, and then to perform glimpses of these lives to others in order to motivate some change of thought or behaviour. Art, after all, according to playwright Tony Kushner, 'is not merely contemplation, it is also action, and all action changes the world, at least a little' (cited in Nicholson 2005, p. 8).

The notion of the performative has become widespread in the social sciences and humanities in recent years. We live in the society of the spectacle and in such a society the citizen becomes spectator (Lehmann 2006, p. 183). The 'metaphor of theatricality' infiltrates almost any attempt to understand social actions and conditions; this is perhaps unsurprising in a world that is 'highly self-conscious, reflexive, obsessed with simulations and theatricalizations in every aspect of its social awareness' (Carlson, cited in Thrift and Dewsbury 2000, p. 419). Erving Goffman, Victor Turner and others have emphasised the theatrical nature of politics and the media, and of social life more generally, arguing that 'the ritualistic staging of successful, winning performances does increasingly matter, with consequences that could not be more real and important' (Szakolczai 2007, p. 4). It is thus vital to acknowledge that arts-based research with communities using theatrical and performance-led methods happens within these wider social and political performances, and 'the limits of the former can only be understood within a close analysis of the framework of the latter' (Thompson 2009, p. 8).

The various performative methods discussed in this chapter are united by a desire to engage an audience and often actively involve them so that they become participants rather than spectators. They are embodied methods (Pelias 2008) and as such they often involve the understanding that knowledge begins from the body (Shapiro 1999). The body has an energetic, material presence that 'produces knowledge of itself and impacts upon the senses of others' (Shepherd 2006, p. 6). Dwight Conquergood (1991, pp. 180–181), a protagonist of performance ethnography, describes this privileging of the body as 'an intensely sensuous way of knowing' and in opposition to measured, theoretical accounts that repress bodily experience. Embodied sociologists similarly seek out opportunities that give rise to 'affect, interconnection and transformation' rather than pursuing 'ideals of analytical tidiness, and objective, rational and scientific protocols' (Inckle 2010, p. 35).

Paying attention to the body, as well as having epistemological consequences, also has implications in terms of emancipation and social change. Any approach committed to human liberation must 'seriously address the body as a site for both oppression and liberation' (Shapiro 1999, p. 18). Bodies are not neutral, but rather are marked by gender, sexuality, ableness, class, race and ethnicity (Pelias 2008, p. 188). Feminist and postmodern theory has paved the way for understanding how the body can be seen as 'the site of culturally inscribed and disputed meanings, experiences, and feelings that can, like emotion, be mined as sources of insight and subjects of analysis' (Fonow and Cook 2005, p. 2216). Peter McLaren (1999, p. viii) expresses it thus:

No matter how distant, removed, and powerless human beings feel in relation to the complexity of contemporary social and economic life, they carry the mega- and microstructures of social life in the machinery of their flesh, in the pistons of their muscle, in the furnaces of their guts, and in the steely wires of their tendons.

Performance often requires embodying the experiences of somebody else. This process results in a way of knowing the other 'that is both rigorous and engaged' (Conquergood 1993, p. 339). In methods such as forum theatre that involve the audience, participants draw on their own corporeal experiences and employ their own bodies to 'intervene in, disrupt or engage productively … opening new research pathways' (Parker-Starbuck and Moch 2011, p. 214). Even in more traditional theatre, audience reaction can be seen as embodied. A presence or energy is manifest in a successful performance which produces a 'special theatrical life' (Schechner 1985, p. 10). An audience's bodily response to tension or dramatic action can be visibly observed: from a leaning forward in one's seat (Shepherd 2006, p. 8) to an overt 'muscular empathy' that happens during sporting performances. As Shepherd (2006, p. 74) points out, 'There's no rational need for the upper body to rise as your team gets closer to the opposing goal'. These responses tend to be collective and quite distinct from the rather more passive act of viewing film or television where any affective response would be an individual one (Schechner 1985, p. 11).

The chapter argues that performance can engage spectators 'emotionally, viscerally and intellectually'. Moreover, it 'opens up multiple, nuanced and often contradictory spaces for consideration and reflection' (Grehan 2009, p. 2). Performance thus holds much radical potential and hope, yet at the same time it 'also holds just as much power to reinforce dominant power structures' (Snyder-Young 2010, p. 891). Certainly, 'an agenda of change set from the outside is more often an imposition than an act of liberation' (Thompson 2003, p. 41). Moreover, even if participants are involved in setting the research agenda and their stories are faithfully rendered, the extent to which spectators' empathy can effect change is questionable. For instance, whilst a collective response has power, this 'does not occlude the possibility of alternative individual responses' (Grehan 2009, p. 31). These individual responses need not be 'negative' or reactionary, but still this suggests that the effects of performance are messy and complex.

There are two broad camps that work with dramatic performance as research (Gray 2003). Whilst one has its roots in theatre or performance studies, the other is rooted in ethnography. The section 'Acting out' traces some of this legacy, then moves on to look at examples of 'ethnodrama' which enable discussion of authenticity in performance. The section ends by reflecting on the role of the audience in this process. This raises the question of whether witnessing performed stories of hardship might serve to 'generate a kind of awe and brief sadness that can be talked about on leaving the theatre but then set aside'; empathy does not always translate into action, and thus spectators 'have the potential to be, positioned as "voyeurs" or tourists who are collectors of aesthetic experiences'

(Grehan 2009, pp. 136–137). The subsequent section, 'Watching and waiting', brings to the foreground this association of affective identification with voyeurism. This takes two of Suzanne Lacy's performance art installations, along with a performance ethnography, as illustrative examples. In the section 'Musical interlude', meanwhile, the theme of voyeurism lurks in the background as the spotlight shines on the role of music and dance in social research. These arguably under-used methods might certainly be employed as energetic and showy forms of communication with an audience, but they can conversely enable a quieter opportunity for self-reflection and the development of a more interior knowledge. 'Breathing new life' discusses examples of performance poetry, film and a tongue-in-cheek striptease. Here there is no escape from issues of the spectator's gaze and emphasis is given to the challenges of confronting an audience with uncomfortable messages.

Acting out

Theatre has a long history of 'reflecting upon, interpreting, portraying, and potentially changing certain aspects of the human condition' (Etmanski 2007, p. 105), and remains a dynamic, contemplative and often instructive art form. 'Applied theatre' (see Nicholson 2005; Prentki and Preston 2009; Thompson 2003) encompasses a wide range of practices that take place outside the confines of the traditional playhouse, including theatre for development, theatre in education, community theatre, theatre in prisons and so on. Each approach has its own set of theories and debates, values and aspirations (Nicholson 2005, pp. 2–3). Some of these might be more *overtly* political than others, but that does not mean that they do not all hold inherent potential to create changes in the community (Prentki and Preston 2009, p. 9). Bertolt Brecht has had a huge influence in this field with his theatre based on Marxist ideology that aimed to reveal both the necessity and inevitability of social change (Prentki 2009a, p. 20). Brecht employed the notion of dialectics throughout his work, in order not only to highlight the contradictions of capitalist societies, but also to explore 'the incompatible and the comic' and to delight in 'unresolved confusion' (Willett 1977, p. 85). His *Lehrstücke*, or teaching plays, were musical in origin and designed to teach 'certain broad social and communal virtues' (ibid., p. 116). However, he is best known for his later 'epic' theatre which involved techniques of breaking the 'magic spell' of theatre; 'of jerking the spectator out of his torpor and making him use his critical sense' (ibid., p. 172). Brecht valued spectators' identification with the *performers* of his plays rather than the characters. For Brecht, the act of empathising with the characters was troublingly bound up with bourgeois illusions (Nicholson 2005, p. 74). Brecht's work gained popularity with UK and US audiences in the 1950s, and thus his influence coincided with the experimental activist theatre of the 1960s and 1970s (Prentki and Preston 2009, p. 12).

Brecht's influence can be seen in the work of Augusto Boal, another key figure in applied theatre. Boal requires audience members to identify *as* performers (Nicholson 2005, p. 75), thus taking 'Brecht's exhortation for audiences to identify *with* the performers to its logical next stage'. Boal's work is also indebted to Paulo Freire; the title of his groundbreaking *Theatre of the Oppressed* (1979) pays homage to Freire's *Pedagogy of the Oppressed* (1970). Boal devised a range of techniques for working with marginalised groups, of which forum theatre is perhaps best known. This is an interactive theatre developed from people's experiences of oppression or discrimination. After a brief performance of the issue at stake, a facilitator known as the Joker – a kind of trickster figure – typically engages the audience in discussion. The Joker is thus called because, like the Joker in a pack of cards, the role is a multiple one that may involve being 'supporter, provocateur, interpreter or friend' (Banks et al. 2014, p. 7). The play then resumes, but this time the action is frozen if an audience member, or 'spect-actor' in Boalian terminology, wishes to try out a different version of events. The spect-actor is encouraged by the Joker to take over from the protagonist and act out his or her ideas; to tell a different story.

The erosion of division between audience and performers is particularly important in applied theatre (Nicholson 2005, p. 75) and is what differentiates it from mainstream theatre (Prentki 2009a, p. 19). This also tends to be a feature of ethnographic performance texts. In privileging their audience, performance texts aim to provide insight that will effect instrumental change.

> In the moment of performance, these texts have the potential to overcome the biases of a positivist, ocular, visual epistemology. They undo the gazing eye of the modernist ethnographer, bringing audiences and performers into a jointly felt and shared field of experience.
>
> (Denzin 2003, p. 37)

Omi Osun Joni L. Jones (2006, p. 339) defines ethnographic performance texts as research that is embodied either by the researcher, the fieldwork community, the audience, or any combination of these participants. The 'sensuous detailing' of ethnographic experience is thus 'given flesh'. There is a significant history of performance texts in ethnographic research, not least as a response to the 'textualism' of the earlier generation of ethnographers (Denzin 2003, p. 16). Not only did the emphasis on writing ethnography fail to capture the world as a performance, it also privileged a particular way of knowing:

> Only middle-class academics could blithely assume that all the world is a text because reading and writing are central to their everyday lives, and occupational security.
>
> (Conquergood 2002, p. 147)

Dwight Conquergood was instrumental in redefining the groundbreaking work of Victor Turner and Richard Schechner, who can be regarded as 'founding fathers' of performance ethnography. For Conquergood it was important that performances actively involved researched communities rather than performing stories about their lives. He introduced a Bakhtinian sense of dialogue to the genre (Omi Jones

2006, p. 340), the notion of speaking to and with, rather than about. (He did, however, in his later work acknowledge the power imbalances that remain inherent in this way of working.) Contemporary performance ethnography continues to lean towards emancipatory intentions in its desire to tell the stories of the researched from their own perspectives and in their own words to a wide and varied audience (which is likely to include informants of the research). Gone are the authoritative voices of ethnographers, who instead seek to 'realign their work with the complexity of the cultures they seek to portray' (Bagley 2008, p. 68). 'Ethnodrama' is one notable means of attempting such faithful portrayal (Mienczakowski 1996; 2000; Mienczakowski and Morgan 2001). This approach involves drawing on researchers' field notes, interview transcripts or diaries and turning the data into performance. Ethnotheatre (Saldaña 2008; 2011) is a related practice that involves traditional techniques of theatre production to produce a performance based on fieldwork. Other performance texts are more 'messy' (e.g. Denzin 1997; Trinh 1991) and less inclined to faithfully render the words of informants, but rather focus on the complexity of lived experience.

Ethnodrama is a collaborative process that involves the research team and often a professional dramatist. Mienczakowski (2000) has used this approach in health research with effective results. *Busting* describes experiences of alcohol detoxification, whilst *Syncing out Loud* looks at issues around schizophrenia. Johnny Saldaña et al.'s *Street Rat* (2005) presents the findings of a research project with homeless young people through ethnodrama. Through the postperformance discussions that routinely take place, the process can be seen as extending forum theatre (Denzin 2003, p. 28). Ethnodrama formed part of a dissemination strategy in research that I carried out at a Sure Start programme in northwest England. Chapter 6 charts the process of this research which culminated in a series of performances as a way of communicating research findings to a diverse audience that importantly comprised of local families as well as professionals and academics. These included readings of poetry written by local women; screenings of short films; and two short plays, *The Bus Stop* and *The Wizard of Us*. The latter play emerged organically through the research process and was instigated with much enthusiasm by the local families involved (see Chapter 6), whereas *The Bus Stop* is an example of the ethnodrama that, from the very start of the research project, I had resolved to attempt (Figure 5.1). I acknowledge that there lies an irony in my determination to effect this method when participants were initially less than eager, given that ethnodrama offers potential to return 'the ownership, and therefore the power, of the report to its informants as opposed to possessing it on behalf of the academy' (Mienczakowski 1996, p. 255).

The Bus Stop involved a collaboration between a local amateur dramatist, the research team (comprised of local women) and the drama group that was set up as a strand of the research project. The two-act play was constructed from data that the research team had collected through questionnaires and interviews with local mothers. Many of the words spoken in the play were taken verbatim from the interview transcripts and reflected the differing attitudes that participants in

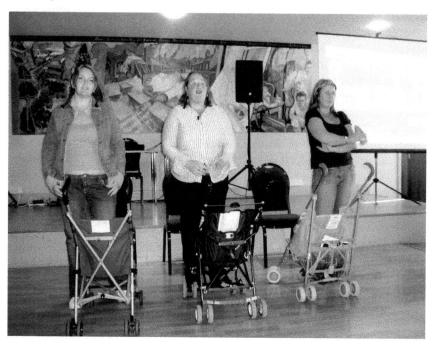

Figure 5.1 Performers in *The Bus Stop* ethnodrama

the research had expressed about Sure Start. In the play, three characters, all mothers of young children, stand at a bus stop. Whilst waiting for a bus (few local families owned their own transport), the women discuss their experiences of motherhood and their interactions with the local Sure Start programme. One character is enthusiastic about the services on offer and encourages the second to attend as they share their experiences of feeling bored and isolated, 'stuck at home with the kids'. The third woman is vocal about her suspicions of Sure Start and its 'interfering' staff. The second act takes place some months later when the women find themselves together at the bus stop again. The first two women are now both involved with the Sure Start programme and they discuss the ways in which it has impacted on their lives (positively *and* negatively). The third woman remains unconvinced.

The drama was undeniably successful in relaying the stories told through the course of the research. The actors were all local women and mothers of young children. They brought their own children's pushchairs as props and spoke with the distinctive regional accent. In these ways they embodied the interview data in a way that I have always maintained is 'authentic' (e.g. Foster 2009). Indeed, one of the actors pointed out that the script could have been a conversation that she had actually had 'in real life'. There was a sense then of listening in or eavesdropping on local women's chat, and the play held the audience's rapt attention. However, this notion of authenticity is perhaps over-reliant on an untroubled notion of voice. As discussed in Chapter 3, the extent to which voices can be understood as authentic rather than as complex constructions influenced by the research process – and certainly by wider social and political factors – is debatable. The work aimed to challenge the way that working-class mothers are marginalised and viewed in a particular, negative, way (see Foster 2015). However, nowhere did the play address the layers of complexity and the discrimination that are involved in the construction of these experiences and the choices that women make. Had we incorporated a post-performance discussion (as Mienczakowski and others advocate), some of these complexities might have been teased out, or at least acknowledged. The lack of engagement with the audience on this occasion meant that the play acted as a mirror held up to the research stories, without any attempt to theorise them or to explore *with* the audience the extent to which they identified with the narratives. In this sense the voice that was heard was insufficient; 'too frail to carry the solemn weight of political and theoretical expectation that has been laid upon it' (MacLure 2009, p. 97). (The play also lacked the sparkle and humour that characterised *The Wizard of Us*. This more anarchic performance came closer to Denzin's [2000, p. 258] vision of an interpretive methodology for a radical democratic social justice, in that it attended to the researched community 'with its own symbolism, mythology, and heroic figures', drawing on 'vernacular, folk, and popular culture forms of representation'.)

Julie Salverson (2001, p. 123) certainly agrees that an over-reliance on the 'authentic' words of storytellers in a performance is at the expense of theorising experiences which are presented at face value or as 'mirrorings'. She also suggests that it might be at the expense of aesthetics in that it limits possibilities. Salverson's focus is on performances of violence and pain. She reflects on having viewed performances that, whilst aiming to highlight issues of travesty and injustice, are almost erotic in their delivery; stories that simplify the relationships between 'victims, villains and heroes'. It follows that the responses of the viewer are also limited and inadequate. A more ethical approach would acknowledge the complexities of relationships between pedagogical approaches, theatrical form and the responses of the audience or participants. This arguably requires a light touch whereby 'obligation [is] traced but not required' and 'meanings [are] touched but not pinned down' (ibid., p. 125). Performance would act as a 'doorway' or instrument of encounter, with the goal not just of empathising but of attending and even witnessing.

Watching and waiting

Suzanne Lacy's feminist performance art provides an interesting example of possibilities of challenging the voyeurism of the spectator when addressing experiences of violation. Lacy has long understood the practice of making art as a process of research (Lacy 2010, p. 321). *She Who Would Fly* was produced in 1977 as part of the series 'Three Weeks in May' which looked at the extent of reported rapes in Los Angeles. This performance installation involved a sequence of events (Video 8). The first involved inviting people who had experienced rape into the gallery to share their stories. The narratives were written out and pinned on the gallery walls. A group of Lacy's students then told their stories of violation, and they also took part in a ritualised event which saw them coating their bodies with red dye and then eating a meal together. For the third stage of the work, visitors were invited to enter the small, contained space of the gallery three or four at a time. This was an intimate space which not only contained all the accounts that had been relayed about rape, it also had on display a lamb carcass with white turkey wings attached which appeared to be struggling to leave the ground. Lacy meant for this to be a metaphor for violence, symbolising the way that when a woman is raped her consciousness attempts to take off and separate from the body and the brutality of what is happening to it. Viewers found themselves voyeuristically consuming women's experiences of violation. Yet as they looked, most people would start to become aware of being watched. They might hear the noise of breathing in the silence of the gallery space, or be conscious of the gallery's spotlight shining down on them. This would lead them to look up and see that above the door, perched on a ledge, were four of the students, crouched naked and bird-like, anointed with red dye, looking intently at the spectators below.

The jolt of shock that spectators might feel does not equate to the experience of rape, but it is still a powerful and thought-provoking reversal of the subject of the gaze. However, it arguably lacks the engagement between the viewer and viewed that can lead to deepening awareness. In Lacy's later work, which is still concerned with looking and perceiving, there is an increased emphasis on dialogue. Reflecting on one such project, *Code 33: Emergency, Clear the Air* which took place in October 1999, Lacy draws parallels between her work (and that of feminist performance art more generally) and Boal's *Theatre of the Oppressed*. This work was not influenced by Boal – indeed, Lacy credits Allan Kaprow (see Kaprow 2003) for the shape that her work took – but there are significant points of comparison. In the same way that Boal called for a theatre outside of the playhouse, Lacy (and other feminist artists) began to work outside of the gallery, engaging the public in projects that were activist and dialogic and which often shared an interest with *Theatre of the Oppressed* in terms of the politics of perception. Boal (cited in Lacy 2010, p. 278) gives an example of the relationship of the gaze to oppression, one he observed in the Satrouville mental hospital:

> I was surprised at the expression in [the nurses'] faces which changed according to whom they were looking at. When their eyes met mine, they were polite but when they looked at a kid, they became authoritarian, severe, and tough ... Let's assume that ... I was taken for a sick person. How long would I have been able to stand it?

Code 33 involved assembling 150 teenagers, 100 policeman and 50 neighbourhood representatives in a series of talks on the roof of a downtown car park in Oakland,

California (see Roth 2001 for a detailed account). This dramatic grand finale, the space floodlit by car headlights and stage lights as well as the spotlight from a police helicopter circling above, was the culmination of much labour. Lacy spent a year working with young people in Oakland, many of whom went on to take part in the performance, playing the roles they assumed in everyday life (much like in Boal's theatre). During this period of time, Lacy notes a shift in the gaze with which she viewed the young people. Initially she was attracted to the aesthetic vision of the 'hooded sweatshirts, baggy pants, and loud theatrical street discourse' from which she was squarely excluded (Lacy 2010, p. 279). However, as she came to know many of the young people she realised that she 'no longer visually noted grey, hooded sweatshirts' but found herself 'unconsciously peering *inside* the hoods' to see if she recognised the wearer; rather than note the pattern and colour of police cars as they passed, she would examine their occupants. Through the course of the research, Lacy brought young people and police officers together in a series of conversations about their lives. Whilst these conversations were on a much more modest scale than those that took place during the lavishly orchestrated grand finale, participants noted how their perceptions of each other shifted through the process. Again this links with Boal's work: 'in both there is a metaphoric situating of the individual such that his or her body, or presence, challenges stereotypical perceptions and categories' (ibid.). The gaze of the audience is key in terms of redefining public actions as art. Lacy also notes that Boal's social justice goals were configured as an aesthetic strategy.

> The aesthetic space is the creation of the audience: it requires nothing more than their attentive gaze in a single direction for this space to become 'aesthetic', powerful, 'hot', five-dimensional ... The objects no longer carry out their usual daily signification, but become the stuff of memory and imagination ... Every tiny gesture is magnified, and the distant becomes closer.
>
> (ibid., p. 275)

If the audience contributes to the aesthetics of performance, then so do aesthetics 'play a crucial role in determining the content of a piece of theatre and further, what that content might mean in the collective and individual understanding of an audience' (Prentki 2009a, p. 19). However, there is a tendency for applied theatre to marginalise the aesthetic in favour of the 'applied' nature of the work. Wiltshire and Hine's (2014) play *Project XXX* focuses on issues related to young people's sexuality and internet pornography. The writers had worked with groups of young people in order to gather their experiences and understandings of sex and pornography, and during the process had discovered gaps in young people's knowledge of contraception. They attempted to incorporate a message in the play regarding contraception, but this did not work with the aesthetics of the play; rather it came across as a public health announcement, according to the writers (during after-show conversation). However, they remained slightly uncomfortable that the artistic merit of the play was at the expense of an opportunity to educate.

Omi Jones (2002) also plays with aesthetics, the gaze and embodied knowing in her performance ethnography *Searching for Osun*. Replete with objects, costumes, rituals and practices that Omi Jones brought back to the USA from her fieldwork with the Yoruba in Nigeria, *Searching for Osun* assumes that people learn through participation and that to understand a culture 'they must put aspects of that culture onto their bodies' (Omi Jones 2002, p. 7). The performance therefore actively involved its audience in a range of activities. It took place in a gallery in Austin, Texas, where Omi Jones loosely marked out various performance areas: The Children's Area, The Market, The Divining Area, The Food Area and The Drumming Area. Eight performers, including one child performer who ran 'endless errands' for her elders, took on a range of roles which involved them interacting spontaneously with the audience as well as each other. For instance one performer was tasked with welcoming people and, in this role, might praise the beauty of their spirit or pray for their prosperity through improvised, repetitive poetry.

As well as sharing knowledge of a culture, the work was also intended to acknowledge ethical and political dilemmas that ethnographic fieldwork and representation raise. Omi Jones had videos and audios playing of 'real' Yoruba culture that she had collected through fieldwork, as a way of highlighting the constructed nature of any representation. She was also concerned with her own subjective role in the whole process, her role as 'interpreter' of a culture, and the way that she situated herself in the performance. One of the two overlapping research questions centred on the identity construction of an African American in Nigeria. (The other explored the nature of Osun.) An earlier reincarnation of the performance ethnography gave much more emphasis to Omi Jones' own experiences. It laboured the 'travel tropes of arrival, disorientation and departure' and in so doing began to 'obscure the ethnographic details of Yoruba life'. This was not just problematic in terms of educating the audience; Omi Jones felt that *she* was not learning anything new about herself or the Yoruba through this work. In contrast, the improvisational nature of *Searching for Osun* allows for new understandings, through 'each audience encounter or each unrehearsed conversation with a performer'. Omi Osun Jones has continued to develop this embodied, performative work. More recently she has spoken about what embodiment tells us about Blackness, and has challenged audience members to think about the histories that are brought to their looking (Video 9). This also poses a challenge to the academy in which she, as a Black academic, is situated: 'In the academy we act like we don't have bodies, but we do!' This exclamation is accompanied by a celebratory, gyrating dance to the beat of drums played by a live musician.

Musical interlude

Dance and music offer exhilarating possibilities of taking 'a journey into ourselves – an inquiry of body and soul' (Snowber 2002, p. 21). This suggests a self-reflective process and so researchers or research participants might be encouraged to explore these methods without necessarily involving a wider audience. There is potential here to listen to what Lisa Mazzei (2009, p. 46) terms the 'silent voice'; that voice that 'resists classification and a desire for "authenticity"'. The medium of dance, for instance, requires paying attention to unspoken 'bodily nuances and cues that come to us each day' (Snowber 2002, p. 22). These might include 'the tension in our shoulders, the flurry in our chests, the grimace on our faces, the joy rising up in our torsos, the sense of expectancy we feel when there is a new possibility' (ibid.). Recognising this body knowledge can awaken new insights (Cancienne and Snowber 2003, p. 248). Snowber provides the example of a dance she developed and performed with a chair after a knee injury prevented the unsupported movement she had been used to. Through the process of listening to her body and discovering its abilities and limitations, Snowber found that she started to develop her thinking about paradox and the very notion of limits:

> I have not always thought of limits as places of possibilities but places of obstacle, something to be jumped, danced, or skipped over. I certainly could not have seen how a place of extension and openness could be sustained and fostered by a limit. The constraint of having a knee injury motivated me to use the chair as a support. What emerged from this experience was an entirely new movement language, which I perhaps never would have found otherwise.
> (ibid., p. 247)

The body, and the dance, thus become the teacher. Ordinary, everyday acts are the subject. Understood in this way, dance might also be viewed as offering the possibility of resistance. Dance is oppositional 'to the dominant ideology for women, because dancing is about taking up space, defying stasis, being strong, and bending of the "normal" images and relationships of what "gendered" human beings can be and do' (Shapiro 1999, p. 6). Snowber's piece *The Zen of Laundry* (Video 10) speaks to the expectations placed on women's daily lives. 'I am doing so many things at the same time', Snowber declares. As she repeatedly spins, bends and stretches she lists the chores that so many women (particularly mothers) are expected to do as 'life goes on and on and on and on'. Partnered by a laundry basket for much of the dance, Snowber begins to repetitively fold the garments within it. With this 'zen' practice of continual folding comes the dawning recognition that the expectations the narrator has of her life need 'loosening'. Movements become ever more expansive and the garments are shaken out of the strictures of their folds. This recalls Robert Linhart's (1981, cited in Highmore 2002a, p. 160) experience of working on a factory assembly line, making the same movements over and over:

> But life kicks in and resists. The organism resists. The muscles resist. The nerves resist. Something, in the body and the head, braces itself against repetition and nothingness. Life shows itself in more rapid movements, an arm lowered at the wrong time, a slower step, a second's irregularity, an awkward gesture, getting ahead, slipping back, tactics at the station; everything, in the wretched square of resistance against the empty eternity of

the work station, indicates there are still human incidents, even if they're minute; there's still time, even if it's dragged out to abnormal lengths. This clumsiness, this unnecessary movement away from routine, this sudden acceleration, this soldiering gone wrong, that hand that has to do it all again, the man who makes a face, the man who's out of step, this shows that life is hanging on. It is seen in everything that yells silently within every man on the line, 'I'm not a machine!'

It is that which is 'normally focal to us', indeed those things that are most common to us, that needs our 'ongoing poetic disruption' (Wiebe and Snowber 2011, p. 110). Dance, understood as 'a sensuous feeling form', can be 'literally and evocatively one of the most moving methods' (Cancienne and Bagley 2008, p. 171), freeing us from stale, unproductive thinking and doing.

A rather different use of dance in the research process may involve the interpretation and performance of research data that has been collected by more conventional means. Mary Cancienne and Carl Bagley have undertaken several collaborations whereby Cancienne dances Bagley's data (Bagley and Cancienne 2002; Cancienne and Bagley 2008). This has included an educational research data set concerned with the impact of school choice on families with children with special educational needs. Cancienne portrayed the ordeal of making this choice through a mime involving walking on a tightrope.

> *She loses her balance and falls and, with her hands and feet, walks backwards frantically, breathing heavily, and then suddenly stops, faces the audience, and with a look of fraught anguish, says,* 'It was a nightmare, literally.'
> (Cancienne and Bagley 2008, p. 180; italics in the original)

Dance is used here as an alternative form of communication with an audience, and this is engaging and exciting, evocative and thought-provoking in ways that a written research report is unlikely to be. However, like other methods of performance, it also involves those sticky issues pertaining to identification and interpretation, which are impossible to avoid for long and which walk a very fine line between being problematic and useful in terms of promoting social justice. As Leela Fernandes (2003, p. 90) notes, 'there is no objective, measurable distance between voyeurism and witnessing; the distinction is qualitative and subtle'.

Music might also be used as a form of communication in research and thus offer potential opportunities for learning and resistance. Song, for instance, is one of the oldest ways of musical communication and has had a major role to play in social justice histories. Like the examples of dance above, there is also something inherent and intangible in music that offers a means of self-reflection or a shared understanding that cannot be verbally expressed, a possibility for attending to 'the ephemeral, to the ebb and flow of lived and researched experience' (Bresler 2008, p. 234). Interestingly, in indigenous cultures, 'place' can be defined by spirit and song as much as physical territories (Smith 2012, p. 129). Smith quotes an

Aboriginal friend saying that 'we sing the land into existence'. In this sense, 'the impact of song goes far beyond the power of the word; it also speaks to the soul' (Albergato-Muterspaw and Fenwick 2007, p. 151).

Francesca Albergato-Muterspaw and Tara Fenwick (2007, pp. 155–158) look at aspects of musical knowing related to participation in a community choir which, as well as communicating political messages, can be seen as bringing participants together. Members of the choir are united through 'breath, vibration, language and synchronous connection with others' (ibid., p. 148). Music can be understood as inclusive and holistic in the way that different tempos and rhythms elicit different emotional and physiological responses with a 'palpable affect on the body' (ibid., p. 150). Albergato-Muterspaw and Fenwick provide examples of a variety of community choirs and their mission statements. Some focus on promoting social change, others on celebrating cultural diversity. Notre Dames des Bananes is a left-wing radical choir in Alberta that sings on picket lines, at political rallies and community events. Whilst some of its songs are written by group members, others are classic labour songs. The choir can be heard performing the powerful anti-war song *Johnny I Hardly Knew Ye* (Video 11). What is important here is not whether or not the choir wrote the song, but the process of coming together to 'plumb the spirit of a song's message' (ibid., p. 158).

Diane Austin and Michele Forniash (2006) distinguish between research studies that incorporate music in the presentation of data, and studies in which the results themselves are a piece of music that has been created from the research process. Austin's research at Alcoholics Anonymous provides an engaging example of the latter. She spent four months attending a weekly open AA meeting. The participants varied from week to week, and Austin was able to amass a large collection of stories and to explore her reactions to these in a reflective journal. This took the form of notes, memos, poetry, song, metaphor and collage. She also carried out interviews with group members. The data was worked into a musical production, *Grace Street*. It opens with a rap by one of the male characters:

> The pain, the pain
> Hey, it's driving me insane
> I'm sitting here and watching
> My life go down the drain
> I'm drugging and I'm drinking
> My thinking is stinking
> And the ship I've been on has hit
> And I'm sinking

(Austin and Forniash 2006, p. 464)

Rap is just one genre of music in the production. A different male character sings the blues; a female character sings the plaintive song, *Somewhere in the Darkness*, devised for the production from the research process. Musical structure, along with the words of songs, is important in terms of communicating to listeners. The audience will ideally be swayed by an immersion in sound that 'moves emotions of outrage and longing, rouses critical awareness at deep levels of being, and opens imaginations to new possibilities' (Albergato-Muterspaw and Fenwick 2007, p. 158). Whilst Austin and Forniash (2006) describe mixed reactions to their production, they celebrate the ability of the musical performance to *breathe life* into the research findings.

Breathing new life

Music and dance are very much about rhythm and breath. Poetry, particularly when it is performed, is also centred on breath; this 'shapes the rhythm, intonation, speed, and resonance of sound' (Cancienne and Snowber 2003, p. 249). Leggo, in his work on knowing through poetry, describes rhythm as

> balance, the flowing of blood, breath, breathing, not breathtaking but breathgiving. Rhythm is the measure of speech, of the heart, of dancing, of the seasons, knowing the living word, the energy of language to inscribe, inspirit hope, even in the midst of each day's wild chaos.

> (2008, p. 167)

Attention to the rhythm of the breath is a powerful way of focusing the mind on the knowledge communicated by the body (Cancienne and Snowber 2003, p. 249). It is also a significant way of relaxing, of tuning out the chatter of the mind, and this is important in terms of listening to others. Walter Benjamin (1969/2006, p. 367), reflecting on the conditions necessary for storytelling to flourish, concludes that the 'more self-forgetful the listener is, the more deeply is what he listens to impressed on his memory'. He describes how the rhythm of traditional work, of weaving and spinning, nurtured the art of listening to and re-telling stories. Listening is an 'interiorising experience, a gathering together, a drawing in' (Conquergood 1991, p. 183). This is in contrast to observation, the gaze that 'sizes up exteriors'.

Caroline Hodges et al.'s (2014) performance poetry project requires attentive listening to hear its participants' words which are often indistinct and laboured, but doing so can bring rich rewards. It is interesting to view the work in light of Mazzei's (2009, p. 50) campaign for a 'move towards a refutation of a normative and "understandable" voice in pursuit of a troubled and difficult to pin down voice'. Drawing on Hélène Cixous' (2007) writing, Mazzei describes this as 'a voice that is speech/silence rather than speech or silence'. This is an unconventional voice that is worthy of attention. Being open to others in this way requires artfulness, 'a listening for the background, the half-muted' (Back 2007, p. 8).

The project involved a collaboration between university academics and a local residential and day school for young people with physical disabilities or complex medical conditions. A series of participatory performative poetry workshops was provided for a group of the young people (aged 14–20) to explore their experiences of being disabled and how disability is understood (or more often misunderstood) within society. These were facilitated by two professional performance poets along with two academic researchers, the school's drama teacher and support staff (Hodges et al. 2014, p. 1095).

The project's title, *Seen But Seldom Heard*, refers to the fact that, alongside typically not being listened to, marginalised groups are also at risk of being subjected to a voyeuristic gaze (Video 12). Through directly addressing an audience via performance, the young people aimed to confront this voyeurism and to raise awareness and understanding of disability. Hodges et al. (2014, p. 1098) attribute this active involvement of the research participants in the planning and delivery of the performances as helping to avoid patronising them or subjecting them to an intrusive gaze. However, they acknowledge that a fine line remains between such confrontations and the encouragement of voyeurism. Sheila Preston draws attention to some of the complex issues inherent in such a debate. She notes that the need to challenge society and its marginalising, hegemonic discourses has to be weighed up with the need to protect people's right 'to speak *or* not speak in private or public' (2009, p. 68). Even with careful handling, representations 'carry their own political significance and resonance in the broader socio-political sphere' and as such they are 'constantly vulnerable to appropriation and redefinition' (ibid., p. 65).

There is little doubt that the subject of the performance poetry project is an important one that holds radical possibilities. It is less of a certainty that the research will not become commodified. However, this is a risk for any research (see Chapter 7). In terms of personal risk, Hodges et al. (2014, p. 1098) note that the young people were able to anticipate and deal with reactions to their performances by drawing on the strategies that they had developed to deal with the day-to-day discrimination they faced. In this regard, the researchers were able to learn from the participants. This added another facet to a complex role for the researchers which included 'event organiser', 'community development worker', 'performance curator', 'PR/promotion' and 'arts advocates' (ibid., p. 1101).

For the People Who Stare (in Hodges et al. 2014, p. 1096; see Video 13) is an example of poem devised and performed by the group:

For the People Who Stare ('The Poetry Sensations')

Get to know the person you're staring at.
What's your problem?
What's your problem?
Try to step into my shoes.
Don't. It makes me scared.
It makes me feel sad.
Everyone is different but judgments take over.
I can't do anything about it.
People are always scared of what's different.
You are disabled to me. I am disabled to you. We are both aliens on this world.

I am crazy but I'm just me, don't look at my wheelchair.
I am open like a magic door.
I am pretty white teeth but yellow on the inside.
I am an actor, gifted with every emotion.
I am a titanium spine worth thousands on Ebay.
I am my own person.
I am a unique cloud, always different every-day.
I am Sean the funny sheep.
I am a football Nickipedia.
I am full of a thirst for knowledge. I want to see a change for the better.
I am everything that I am, I can't change. I wouldn't change it for the world.

Whilst Hodges et al. (2014) claim that the poetry enabled these participants' voices to be heard, it is the performances that breathe life into the participants' words and shape them in ways that draw attention to their unconventional, challenging speakers. This is not just about 'voice'; there is power in the determination and passion with which the words are formed and articulated, and the weight of the worldly, embodied experience behind them. The text itself is arguably less enlightening than the way it is articulated. It is thus frustrating, as Dani Snyder Young (2010, p. 889) points out, that the academy remains text-centric twenty years on from Conquergood's (1991) call for performance to be recognised as a legitimate and scholarly form of representation. However, the growth in video technology and platforms such as YouTube provide an invaluable resource for sharing material and capturing some of the essence of a performance. Hodges et al. (2014, p. 1097) also found that they were able to incorporate film footage of participants writing and performing their work *into* live performances. This worked well for those participants whose difficulties with communication, or geographical locations, meant that they were not able to take part in the live event.

The use of film is also a crucial component of Trish Hafford-Letchfield et al.'s (2010) performance project, *RUDE (Rude Old People)*. This worked with older people to explore intimacy and sex in later life. The project aimed to challenge marginalising, ageist views and to promote the importance of sex and intimacy in terms of older people's well-being and quality of life. Hafford-Letchfield et al. argue the importance of this issue in terms of social work education because, although it is congruent with social work ethics and values, the profession tends to neglect everyday sexuality outside deviant or medical discourses. It thus 'makes pathological what is a basic human need by denying acknowledgement of an individual's culture and identity' (ibid., p. 606). The *RUDE (Rude Old People)* project involved a collaboration between a social work department at a university in the UK and an older people's theatre group. A number of young students were involved in the project and the theatre group brought in independent film-makers in order that the performances devised through a series of workshops could be captured on film. There were opportunities for participants to be involved in the process of writing, directing and filming, and a blog was established for people to reflect on their experiences of the research.

A range of performative methods were used to collect and disseminate data. These included dance 'to a pulsating heartbeat rhythm', role plays, acted out scenarios, stand up comedy and poetry. In all, seventeen video clips were produced from these performances to be used for learning and teaching. Video clips were enhanced by the use of creative editing techniques in an attempt to further provoke reflection in the viewer. For instance, a role play of an assessment for care services incorporates pauses so that viewers are given opportunity to consider the dialogue and other elements of this (potentially marginalising) process. Voiceover recordings enable the viewer to hear what the characters are thinking and to 'consider what is really going on in the scenario other than what we see' (Hafford-Letchfield et al. 2010, p. 609). One of the most challenging of the clips involves an older woman unravelling a red silk sheet wrapped around her naked older body to the show tune *Big Spender* (Figures 5.2, 5.3 and 5.4). Viewers are drawn in to the theatrical striptease and required not only to confront the provocative performance, but also to face their own attitudes towards older women and possibly their fears of the ageing process. The project thus plays with ideas of voyeurism, identification and difference, and actively brings together young and older people 'rather than talking from the safety of their own practice or culture' (ibid., p. 616). The use of humour helps stop the project from straying into the 'earnest' or 'worthy' territory of some projects that attempt to address social justice issues. Laughter releases some of the tension that the performances build, and lends levity to a troublesome and testing issue.

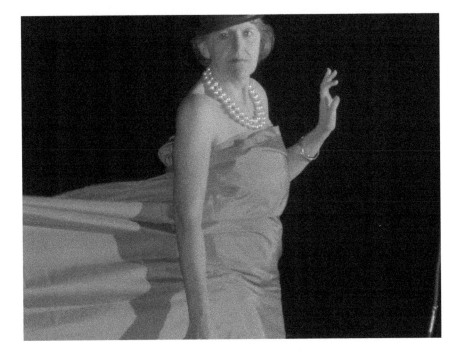

Figure 5.2 Caption on next page

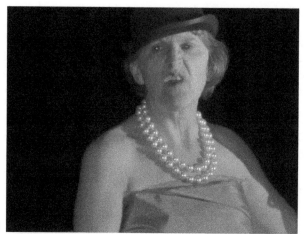

Figure 5.3

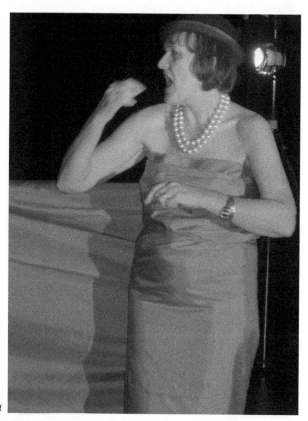

Figure 5.4

Figures 5.2, 5.3 and 5.4 'Hey', 'Big', 'Spender'

Source: Images from the *RUDE (Rude Old People)* project (Hafford-Letchfield et al. 2010). Reproduced with permission.

Conclusion

Performative methods offer stimulating, engaging ways of presenting research data and also of creating new knowledge in the process. This is not a straightforward process, however, and it is important not to be swayed by the appeal of dazzling emancipatory claims, of data dressed up in spangles. Methodological conundrums do not disappear when research data is performed and should not be glossed over. Dilemmas over 'authentic' voice, power dynamics and representation persist and require acknowledgement. There is also a persistent tension in terms of the relational dynamics of performance. Salverson (2001, p. 119) relays the story of a *Theatre of the Oppressed* workshop she attended. At the end of the session the organiser asked the participants to hold hands and declare 'We are from near, we are from far. We are one!' Salverson found herself unable to repeat this glib statement, but also felt unable to voice her reluctance for not doing so. Reflecting on this incident, Salverson thinks about those relationships with people who are *unlike* ourselves. She notes the tendency of theatre based on personal testimony (in this case of experiences of violation and violence) to consume the other person and reduce them to the terms of the theatre maker. This involves a distortion of relationships and also a loss of potential in terms of the learning that could be gained. Salverson instead seeks 'a contact that lets us come together differently and binds me deeply to another without our collapsing either the "I" or the "other" into a totalising "we"' (ibid., p. 120).

Employed in a sensitive, thoughtful way, performance *can* enable both performers and audience to gain greater insight into their own lives and the lives of others. There is scope to move beyond a voyeuristic gaze, beyond a 'trying on' of other people's lives. Shared verbal, emotional and bodily information 'can create more than a two-way exchange of facts; it can generate a third space in which something new is co-constructed and realized' (Sharma et al. 2009, p. 1648). The generation of this 'third space' can even go as far as to be seen as a soulful encounter. Certainly Walsh et al.'s (2015) volume *Arts-based and Contemplative Practices in Research and Teaching: Honoring Presence* draws attention to the spiritual dimension of art practices and collaborative, mindful, compassionate ways of working, which might act as 'gateways into "other" ways of becoming, knowing and not knowing' (p. 8). The very act of pausing and listening carefully to others is a crucial way of developing understanding, 'spiritual' or otherwise. Similarly, our own bodies might have messages for us if we are able to quieten our thoughts and attend to meaningful 'echoes, silences, yawns and sighs' (Snowber 2002, p. 22).

There is much scope in collaborative arts-based working to explore this sensuous, bodily knowing. The following chapter examines ways in which this was attempted in my Sure Start research. This project was discussed above in relation to my deployment here of ethnodrama and the concerns it raised over authenticity and voice. Chapter 6 provides a much more detailed look at the research and in doing so weaves in a discussion of bodies and embodied knowing in relation to the 'carnivalesque' and a process of inquiry that aims to challenge the status quo.

6 Case study

'They're not like us real mums – are they?'

This chapter describes the process of carrying out a collaborative arts-based research project with poor working-class mothers at a Sure Start programme in the UK. Sure Start is a government-funded initiative that works with children under the age of five and their families with the aim of reducing health and social inequalities. On the surface a useful and supportive initiative, Sure Start is underscored by a neoliberal agenda whereby scrutiny of working-class family life has dramatically intensified, and blame for social ills – such as poverty and crime – is frequently apportioned on individual parents (and more often than not on mothers rather than fathers) (De Benedictis 2012). The exploitative and oppressive nature of such an ideology is a general argument of this book that received elaboration in Chapter 2. That discussion was woven together with motifs of the circus and carnival, highlighting the illusory nature of much of neoliberal rhetoric. These motifs have subsequently made regular appearances throughout the book in order to draw attention to ambiguity, absurdity and possibilities of transformation in the process of knowledge production in neoliberal society. In this chapter, the Sure Start research is viewed in terms of a 'carnivalesque' process and in so doing brings together a number of the methodological ideas and concerns that have been raised in the book thus far.

> Carnival is not time wasted but time filled with profound and rich experience.
> (Clark and Holquist 1984, p. 302)

The Russian literary theorist Mikhail Bakhtin developed notions of carnival and the carnivalesque, most notably through his influential work *Rabelais and His World* (1968/1984). This focused on a type of rebellious late medieval and Renaissance folk humour that can be seen to challenge the status quo and temporarily invert established structures of power. Whilst carnival refers to a festival or celebration, often involving costume and masquerade, the concept of the carnivalesque denotes the application of a carnival 'spirit' to a text: 'the carnivalesque provides a mirror of carnival; it is carnival reflected and refracted through the multi-perspectival prism of verbal art' (Danow 2004, p. 4).

The Sure Start research project was not designed with the carnivalesque in mind, yet my prevailing memories of this period of time are of laughter, chaos and subversion. This carnival spirit is 'a life-affirming and life-enhancing' energy, but there lurks simultaneously a darkness and a revolt against accepted values (Danow 2004, p. 1). For all the colour, humour and laughter that saturated our project, there remained the dark shadow caused not only by poverty, but also by inequality and injustice. There are limits to the extent to which collaborative arts-based research can lift such a shadow. The chapter considers these confines through the use of key notions of the carnivalesque, including humour and resistance, and seeks to elaborate on previous discussion of the paradoxical nature of the research process, its triumphs and its flaws. It also considers how *lasting* any transformations that are produced through the research process might be. This discussion, then, also anticipates Chapter 7, which looks at how we might define the successes and failures of collaborative arts-based research for social justice.

The trilogy of chapters, Chapter 3: 'Storytelling', Chapter 4: 'Image and Metaphor' and Chapter 5: 'Performance', have introduced a number of the ideas that are discussed here, and the concept of the 'carnivalesque' enables a further focus on some of the tensions inherent in this way of working. For instance, there is an ongoing concern over the researcher's relationship to 'truth' and notions of challenging the status quo. The section 'Grotesque bodies' draws its title from an important theme of Bakhtin's work in order to convey the way that the poor working classes are portrayed as 'deviant' in our society. It makes a case for research that aims to challenge the voyeuristic gaze that marginalised people are subject to, but acknowledges the difficulty of doing so (a particular focus of Chapter 5). The section 'Making strange' then highlights the inherent tension of attempting to challenge the establishment whilst working within its strictures, a theme that – introduced in Chapter 2 – has been woven through the book. This section also provides background to the various arts-based groups that were set up as part of the larger research project, including creative writing, short-film making and visual arts. The process of establishing these groups enabled us to employ image and metaphor in the research, as advocated in Chapter 4.

The next section, 'Resistance', considers the extent to which the use of these methods in the research process might challenge perceptions of women's lives, whilst acknowledging the risk that they will only serve to reinforce them. This is one of the main concerns of Chapter 3 which, in relation to storytelling, considered the possibility of hearing alternative voices and a change of story from the hegemonic norm. Here, short films and visual art work produced by the Sure Start women act as illustrative examples. The section 'Playing' focuses on the dramatic performances that we worked on both during the research process and as a means of disseminating research findings. It extends the discussion in Chapter 5, in which I introduced my use of ethnodrama in the Sure Start research. 'Paradox' then discusses spectators' reactions to these performances. This section also pays attention to the role of the researcher in collaborative arts-based research and the extent to which the Sure Start research project might be seen as an opportunity to educate its participants as well as its audience.

The chapter weaves together accounts of individuals' experiences and emotions, their creative responses to the research aims, and the social and political context of the project. This is in line with the book's aim of making links between personal, everyday experiences, described through imaginative and evocative mechanisms, and wider social issues. Our descriptions of society – however imaginative – are inseparable from our culture, our values, beliefs and relationships. Moreover, truth claims are 'always pursued within a context of taken-for-granted assumptions' which tend to remain unchallenged within the research process (Witkin 2000, p. 208). For instance, the propensity to assume that those living in poverty are in some way to blame for their destitution serves to detract attention from the wider social issues that *do* have an incredibly large and complex part to play. Thus assistance is provided in maintaining the status quo. The carnivalesque, meanwhile, assists in revealing and disturbing. It is understood that:

> [T]he social world is not a predetermined and 'natural' reality, but one that is shaped by powerful groups. Such a change in perspective is significant for it can embolden those who make this shift to realize that they can have agency working to re-form the social fabric.
>
> (Martin and Renegar 2007, p. 300)

The Sure Start research served to acknowledge the hegemonic social norms which denigrate the poor working class, particularly mothers who are often demeaned (if not demonised) and viewed as 'other'. This denigration happens pervasively through the media, through everyday interactions and also through ideology underlining policy initiatives such as Sure Start. The resulting tensions that this throws up in terms of the Sure Start programme are explored in the chapter, but are exemplified in its title. This refers to a comment made by a member of the programme's staff at the time the research was taking place. It was my son's first day at school and I was discussing how emotional I felt. She agreed that she had had similar feelings when her children started school, unlike the Sure Start mothers, she said, who could not wait to be rid of their progeny: 'They're not like us real mums, are they?'

Grotesque bodies

Sure Start was announced in 1998 by the UK's New Labour government (1997–2010), and paralleled other social investment approaches such as Head Start in the United States and Canada. In establishing links with health, education, employment and social services, it aimed to provide a more cohesive service for children, investing in their well-being now on the understanding that it would 'pay off' as they reached adulthood (Fawcett et al. 2004, p. 4). It was very much the cornerstone of New Labour's pledge to abolish child poverty, and a flagship among a plethora of initiatives targeted toward the family. Delivered through programmes in the more disadvantaged communities of the UK, Sure Start provided a wealth of public meeting spaces, baby and toddler groups, early-years education, health advice (including smoking cessation and healthy eating) and parenting advice in areas which had never before enjoyed such resources. It was, however, underscored by the problematic assumption that poor families need moral instruction on how to raise their children correctly. At the time of writing, the present coalition government appears to be steadily dismantling the initiative, with many centres closing as a result of a lack of ring-fenced funds.

My own involvement with Sure Start began way back in 2001 at a local Sure Start programme in an ex-mining community in the northwest of England, an area of particular economic and social disadvantage. It had an unemployment rate substantially higher than the national average, and markedly low levels of literacy. I set up a weekly two-hour community art group for parents of the young children attending the programme, which explored different forms of art and crafts, from painting to card making to jewellery making (see Chapter 3). Children were looked after in a crèche in the same building so that participants (mothers and grandmothers) were provided with an adult space; a space that was filled much of the time with raucous laughter as we gossiped and bantered. The group was consistently attended by about a dozen women, ranging in age from late teens to early fifties. None of them had easy lives. A number of them were particularly vocal and feisty and talk was comic, bawdy, punctuated with swearing. As well as demonstrating the week's arts and craft activities, I provided coffee and copious slices of buttered toast. Most indulged in this; others had bottles of water with them which I suspected were laced with amphetamines, but I chose to feign ignorance. I remain convinced that this safe, non-judgemental space was nothing but beneficial. It attracted women who did not engage with many, if any, of the programme's other services.

I remain less comfortable with the outings I arranged to several art galleries. Accompanied by our young children, the majority of them in pushchairs, the visits were much enjoyed and provided new experiences for everyone. However, they also attracted a considerable amount of unwarranted attention from the very middle-class public that we encountered. Reactions to the women and their offspring ranged from unwelcoming to thinly disguised disgust. A number of the women were asked to leave one of the art galleries we attended, with claims that the children were being too noisy. This has never been my (middle-class) experience of attending art galleries with children, before or since this period (and we subsequently received a letter of apology when we complained to the gallery in question). The Sure Start mothers dismissed the incident and laughed at the 'snobs' who met us with a plethora of raised eyebrows and stern stares, but I felt responsible and was shaken by these reactions.

My response was no doubt naïve given that I have long held an academic awareness of the ways in which poor working-class mothers are viewed as deviant and as a threat to the social good (Foster 2015), and how they are frequently depicted in our culture as 'grossly repellent' (Skeggs, interviewed by Almack 2003, p. 3). Such performances of class disgust as we experienced have the very significant purpose of asserting middle-class identity. The working class act as a foil or negative reference point (Lawler 2005, p. 442), which serves to affirm the superiority of the middle class. Tyler (2008, p. 22) notes the emphasis that is placed on appearance in terms of depictions of the working class, in particular 'on a perceived excess of (bodily) materiality'. An excessive appearance, an excessive sexuality and excessive fecundity, as opposed to the modest femininity of the middle classes, pose 'a threat to the moral order of Western civilisation' (Skeggs 2004, p. 100). This evokes the 'grotesque body', a key feature of Bakhtin's carnivalesque. This body is excessive, garish and exaggerated: 'We're talking multiple projections, here, spikes, sprouts, boobs, bums ... and there's something archaic behind it all ... Something positively filthy' (Carter 1994, p. 98). Through the arts-based research, employing costume and parody, the Sure Start mothers can be seen to simultaneously embrace and to challenge their physicality. They become the *producers* of spectacle rather than its subjects. There is a question though over whether, for women, the 'real' world is itself 'a place of diversity, of masks and deception' (Webb 1994, p. 304); what does this play acting mean for women who '*already* exist in a duplicitous state of affectation?'

Making strange

The research project emerged through a series of synchronicities. I had just completed a master's degree which focused on emancipatory research practices, when a call came for each local Sure Start programme to evaluate its services. Guidance on this was issued by the National Evaluation of Sure Start (NESS; a team of researchers based at Birkbeck College, London) and it strongly encouraged parental involvement in the process. There was already a significant component of service-user involvement in the design and delivery of local programmes. However, given that the Sure Start initiative is arguably underscored by an assumption that working-class parents lack competence, there exists a 'contradictory conceptualization of parents as both competent and incompetent' (Clarke 2006, p. 717). Should such paradoxes remain untroubled in the research process then, as discussed in previous chapters, there is a danger for collaborative research approaches to actually *promote* hegemonic understandings rather than challenge them.

As a feminist I championed the need to develop a sociology *with* women (Byrne and Lentin 2000, p. 31) and saw myself very much on 'the side' of the mothers at the Sure Start programme. I wanted to provide space for the women I had come to know in the Sure Start community to articulate their experiences, and by raising the status of their understandings to interrupt the dominant ideology surrounding motherhood. I proposed a methodology that I envisaged would enable me to work together with Sure Start parents (fulfilling the Sure Start objectives) but with counter-hegemonic aims. These aims, I suggest here, are carnivalesque in essence. For what else is carnival if not the '"making strange" of hegemonic genres, ideologies, and symbols?' (Gardiner 1992, p. 32). Carnival can thus be employed as a vehicle of social critique (Martin and Renegar 2007, p. 300) in the context of doing social research.

There is much debate around the extent to which this can happen. The liminal freedom that carnival offers in terms of reversing social hierarchies happens within imposed confines. Despite carnival providing the opportunity for subversion, the license for this has to be granted by the authorities (Taylor 2007, p. 18). So was the research governed by official processes and bodies. Funding was provided by the ESRC in the form of a collaborative 'CASE' award,[1] which meant that the Sure Start programme and the university where I was based contributed to the financial arrangements. This enabled me to undertake the research for my Ph.D. The work I produced had to fulfil the requirements of this programme of study as well as meeting Sure Start's needs in terms of the evaluation produced. The project was also governed by research ethics. Funding for the Sure Start programme came through the local health authority (this was not the case for all of the Sure Start programmes); therefore ethical approval was required from the local National Health Service research ethics committee, a lengthy and convoluted process. There is certainly an incongruity in challenging those 'institutional structures, processes and relationships which maintain or foster silence and isolation' when we are situated within them (Maguire 1996, p. 32).

Despite, or perhaps because of, these strictures, the research methodology aimed to provide opportunity for the Sure Start parents to be involved in creating knowledge about themselves and their experiences of living in the local area, parenting (often in poverty) and their interactions with Sure Start. Not least due to the links I had made through the art group, I was able to recruit, train and work with a group of eight women as 'community researchers'. These were all White, working-class mothers of young children involved in the Sure Start programme. The women varied in age; their ethnicity reflected the ethnic make up of the geographical area, which was overwhelmingly White. Six of the community researchers saw out the whole two years of the entirely voluntary project. A number of this core group also became involved in the arts-based methods, as well as collecting data through more traditional methods of questionnaire and interviews.

The aims of incorporating arts-based methods were to enable the participation of a wider group of 'marginalised' people, and to breathe more life into both data collection and the dissemination of findings. A number of groups and activities were put into place at the beginning of the two years of fieldwork (this lengthy stretch of time enabled the ambitious project). These included a short-film making class, a creative writing class, a visual art workshop that took place within the established art group, and a drama group. Suggestions for these particular activities came from Sure Start parents and they proved popular with local people (predominantly mothers, although the creative writing and visual art projects included grandmothers; and the short-film making and drama group attracted two fathers). I collaborated with local artists and venues to provide tuition, and I attended each of the groups on a weekly basis in order to encourage turnout.

A range of data was thus produced during these two years, from interview transcripts to questionnaires, to collage, short film and poetry. Findings were analysed together with the group of community researchers on an ongoing basis and we identified a number of pertinent themes. In addition to a conventional research report for the Sure Start programme, which I wrote and the community researchers 'verified', we disseminated the data through drama. The short film, collage and poetry were already in a format ready for an audience, but the interview transcripts were worked into short plays. The remainder of the chapter discusses the extent to which the knowledge produced during the research project can be seen as fulfilling carnivalesque aims of subverting hegemonic understandings, of liberating 'from the prevailing point of view', offering 'the chance to have a new outlook' and entering 'a completely new order of things' (Bakhtin, cited in Danow 2004, p. 142). When Bakhtin discusses the potential of carnival he is actually 'articulating a theory that is essentially epistemological at base, one that seeks new ways of knowing and new approaches to understanding the world' (Danow 2004, p. 143).

Resistance

If the Sure Start research was to 'liberate from the prevailing point of view' then it needed to resist those dominant ideologies of motherhood that serve to exclude and vilify the working class. There are a number of ways that resistance could be seen to be happening, not just through the research process itself but also through stories of individual acts of defiance reported by research participants. The participatory approach of having the community researchers design research questions and collect data enabled us to elicit these stories. This approach not only allowed for insightful, in-depth interviews to be conducted with mothers accessing the Sure Start programme, it also proved particularly successful in establishing contact with the most 'hard-to-reach' families in the local area who were eligible to access Sure Start but were choosing not to. We used a door-to-door questionnaire survey to look at the reasons for this, visiting mothers who were living in abject poverty in appalling housing conditions, frequently with mental health problems or physical disabilities. Whilst such disabilities certainly did not make it easy for people to access Sure Start's services, one of the most significant barriers in the way of engagement proved to be the profound misgivings families had towards professionals. Such 'deep suspicion and anxieties that parents have towards social workers and child care intervention' (Williams 2004, p. 418) have a long history, which is not surprising given that poor working-class parents have consistently been the targets of much state intervention, monitoring and management. One survey respondent spoke for many when, discussing social services, she declared, 'Don't have no dealings with them at all. Can't stand 'em.' Sure Start workers (most of whom are not professional social workers) were described as 'too official' by one survey respondent, although she was happy to talk to the community researcher: 'You're normal – you're a mum, you've been there.'

   This recalls the title of this chapter, 'They're not like us real mums' and in true carnivalesque spirit represents an inversion of the dominant thinking. In this project, the poor working-class mother is the norm. Middle class values are suspended. This can be seen in the visual arts project which reveals a different picture of poor working-class motherhood. Participants were asked to take photographs of the most meaningful elements of their lives. These were worked into vivid collages with glowing layers of tissue paper and paint (Figure 6.1). Most of the art works contained photographs of smiling and laughing children; one included a large pan of potatoes which the picture's creator told us were for the huge Sunday dinner that the extended family enjoyed every week. Another picture included a garden gate leading to the participant's home. In one interview, a mother had bemoaned the fact that the Sure Start initiative placed too much emphasis on 'the state of your house … whether it looks like a shed or whatever', when 'there's other things that can be counted that have more of a wealth that you can't see'. The flamboyancy of the art works reveals this hidden wealth, the artificiality of the colours arguably holding more resonance and authenticity than judgemental perceptions of outsiders. One of the participants in the art group summed this up: 'These pictures are real – they're about real lives, real families.'

Two of the short films produced by mothers during the course of the research can also be seen to demonstrate resistance to judgemental attitudes in an effort to liberate audiences from tacitly reproducing hegemonic social norms (but see also Chapter 3 for a different take on these narratives). Participants in the short-film making group were asked to film elements of their family life and to consider their involvement with the Sure Start initiative. *A Better Life* and *… My Life … My Family … My Home* were produced by lone mothers who, having overcome a

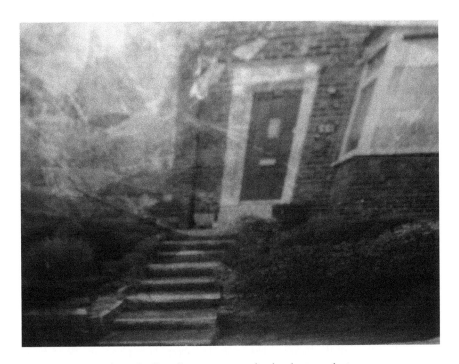

Figure 6.1 Image from the Sure Start programme's visual arts project

history of drug misuse, are living in poverty, very much on the margins of society. The films hum with vibrancy and tongue-in-cheek humour. One woman films her family home, a small house packed with people and clutter. She captures her own mother on film whilst she is pottering in the kitchen with a towel wrapped round her head. Her mother swears fervently as the video camera approaches and we can hear the mischievous chuckles of the film-maker. It then pans to the woman's sister-in-law sprawling on a sofa, pulling faces at the camera. We are taken jerkily upstairs, where we find her brother lying on a bed with his girlfriend, smoking a joint. Back downstairs, the film-maker's two little girls pose and dance; an uncle sweeps one of his tiny nieces up in the air and dangles her by her feet as she squeals. The happy chaos is accompanied by pulsing dance music.

This is all in dramatic contrast to the film-maker's tour of the Sure Start programme which she claims, in a sedate and coherent voice over, has added another dimension to her and her daughters' lives. Whilst this is no doubt the case, her portrayal of the rule-bound, 'sensible' initiative feels rather tongue-in-cheek as she takes the viewer into various offices and puts on an affected accent when describing the work that takes place there. The mother who produced *A Better Life* also credits Sure Start for enhancing her life and 'improving' her parenting. She records wholesome scenes of a country walk in the sunshine with her children, and her own mother baking fairy cakes with the family. However, she has – almost provocatively – also included scenes that do not fit with an idealised middle-class version of motherhood. As with the previous video, there is an abundance of shouting and bad language, and the children are filmed leaping off the garden shed roof into a paddling pool.

Whilst I do not claim these films are typical of poor working-class family life, and elements of them are certainly not to be held up as 'ideal' practice, they do revel in a raucous, chaotic family life and demonstrate the fun that can be had if some of mainstream society's 'rules' (including legal ones surrounding drug use, and the prevalent concern for health and safety) are broken. Seen as carnivalesque, they have the potential of redefining limits of acceptability. Carnival 'is the place for working out, in a concretely sensuous, half-real and half-play-acted form, *a new mode of interrelationship between individuals,* counter-posed to the all-powerful socio-hierarchical relationships of non-carnival life' (Bakhtin 1984, p. 123; italics in the original).

Playing

The carnivalesque is most explicit in the drama element of the research project, which took on a spirited life of its own. The intention was to employ drama to disseminate the findings of the research, influenced particularly by Jim Mienczakowski (1996; Mienczakowski and Morgan 2001) and his work on ethnodrama (see Chapter 5). In order for this to become a possibility, it was necessary to build skills and confidence among the community so they could take part. At the behest of the families that I talked to about these ideas, an after-school drama group was set up in collaboration with a local amateur dramatist who we found through word of mouth. All ages were welcome to the group and soon a range of families was in attendance; sometimes three generations of the same family came. I attended the weekly sessions with my son. After a series of discussions about the group's aims, we decided that we wanted to work on a pantomime. This was the genre of theatre that families were most familiar with, a traditional British form of entertainment that dates back to late Victorian times but remains extremely popular, particularly around the Christmas period. Involving a retelling of a fairytale in a way that incorporates lots of farce, cross-dressing, song and dance, pantomime is also an ideal means through which the carnivalesque can operate, not least through 'the laughter at physical comedy and the grotesque body' (Taylor 2007, p. 18). We scripted *Hansel and Gretel Grow Up*, complete with topical, local jokes. We chose songs and devised dance routines, then spent many happy but extremely chaotic months rehearsing (see Foster 2013). The art group painted backdrops, and parents and grandparents devised costumes (Figures 6.2 and 6.3).

We performed the pantomime in the community and procured a wide audience of local families and professionals. It was well received and participants (including my son and I) were thrilled at the reactions. One Sure Start mother had been reluctant to bring her sons to watch the performance because she worried they would be disruptive. However, she was surprised to find that they were spellbound by the show: 'The boys sat there [throughout the performance] and they never moved'. Another mother who took part in the performance together with her two girls describes the impact the experience had on her daughters:

> Since the panto the kids have been talking amongst themselves, role-playing all the time. They know the lines off by heart. Everything they say is in panto language! They play together more – they've got something to say and act out. They've never got the video [of the panto] off. They show it to everyone. They go to the theatre more now – they love watching plays and pantos.

The plan now, as I had made clear from the start, was for the adult members of the drama group to work on the research data and think of ways of performing

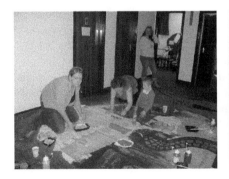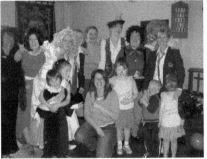

Figures 6.2 and 6.3 Images from the Sure Start programme's preparations for the pantomime

this. To this end, I brought in an expert in forum theatre (see Boal 1979) to provide workshops on this approach. We were encouraged to draw on difficult issues from our own lives, which the Sure Start women found dull and depressing. They wanted to escape from the harsh realities of life, not re-enact them; they wanted to dress up in silly costumes and perform another pantomime.

> In Pantoland
> Everything is grand.

> ... It's a bristling world, in Pantoland, either phallic or else demonically, aggressively female.

(Carter 1994, p. 98)

Shulamith Lev-Aladgem (2000, p. 163) discusses the fact that approaches to acting usually range between two extremes, naturalism and alienation, emphasising either authenticity or artificiality. She discusses a third model of acting, play, 'whereby the performer is playing with acting rather than acting properly'. The '[c]arnivalesque enactment belongs to this family of playing'. It was in this family that the Sure Start mothers desired to be. There followed a lengthy conversation whereby we discussed the mismatch between this and my aim of dramatising the research findings. We started to think about ways of bridging these two very disparate aims and devised *The Wizard of Us*, a short play that tells the stories of the researched through the well known characters from L. Frank Baum's *Wizard of Oz* (see Foster 2013 for more in-depth discussion of this play and excerpts of the script). Dorothy became a young single mother from our ex-mining community. She was, like a significant number of mothers that we spoke to during the course of the research, struggling with postnatal depression. She had experienced a profound sense of isolation after having her baby girl, Toto. This again was a common theme of our research findings. Prior to Sure Start there had been no communal spaces for parents of young children to meet. Even the local park was inaccessible due to broken glass and discarded drug paraphernalia. Dissatisfied with her life, Dorothy sets off to find a better way.

On this journey, Dorothy encounters Scarecrow, Lion and Tinman. She finds Scarecrow smoking a joint, having withdrawn from life. Scarecrow had, like many of our research respondents, been told by parents and teachers that she would never amount to anything. 'They drummed that into us,' said one interview participant, 'that we were like cretins and morons'. Lion lacks confidence to the point that she is unable to leave the house. She spends her days watching daytime television and without any adult company at all. We were told by another interview participant that Sure Start has 'brought my confidence out a bit more and I can talk to people more instead of just sat at home and wouldn't say boo to nobody'.

Tinman has taken time off work to raise his children and has found that he is 'rusty' and doesn't have the qualifications he needs to get back into employment. I was ambivalent about including issues of skill building and employability, not

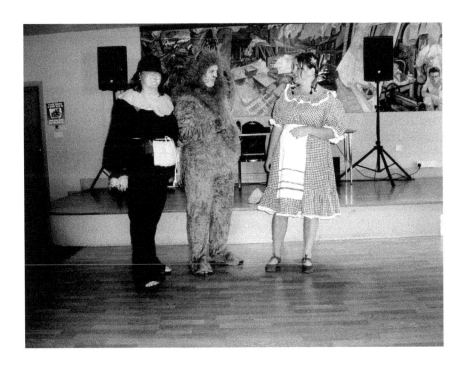

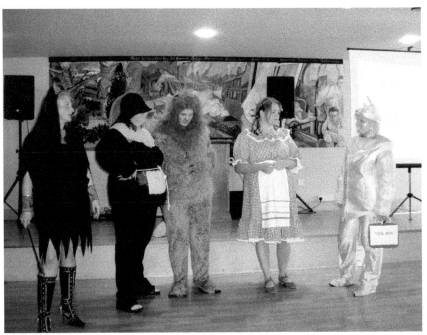

Figures 6.4 and 6.5 Performers in *The Wizard of Us*

least because of the huge emphasis on this as a route out of poverty for families when it is often far from the case. However, the Sure Start parents thought it warranted inclusion in the play. They also overruled me on the conclusion of the play, which ends on a very positive note in terms of the Sure Start initiative. Dorothy and her friends realise that there is help and support for them back in their community and that there's 'no place like home'. This certainly reflected those stories we were told through the research, concerning the benefits that mothers and their children had reaped through the Sure Start programme in terms of making friends and becoming less isolated. There were certainly massive advantages to the initiative. However, the 'happy ending' neglected to address the issues of profound judgement to which – as the research had revealed – the mothers felt subjected.

Paradox

The research project culminated in a dissemination event to which were invited local families, health and social care professionals, academics and Sure Start staff. The event was well attended and comprised dramatic performances (including a short ethnodrama, *The Bus Stop*, discussed in Chapter 5; see also Foster 2012a), as well as poetry readings (see Foster 2007; 2012b for more discussion of poetry in social research) and showings of the visual arts project and the short films (Foster 2009). The event was warmly received by its audience who declared themselves startled by the talents and 'bravery' of the Sure Start mothers involved. One health professional noted that it s '[e]xcellent to see all the talents and strengths of people in the community, who often I see during my work hours, to see another side to their lives was fantastic'. Given that poor working-class mothers are so often viewed as incompetent and lacking, this was a positive reversal. As Pablo Martin and Valerie Renegar (2007, p. 301) stress, 'carnival's particularly ambivalent form of parody serves to reveal that established social structures are constructions that are open to debate, competition, and revision'.

However, at the same time, Sure Start workers were quick to take credit for the mothers' achievements:

> I found the presentation today very moving (can't believe I couldn't stop crying!). I've been a member of staff in the programme virtually from the beginning and am so happy to see the parents ... on that stage today with loads of confidence ... *The Wizard of Us* play was excellent and got loads of messages across. I feel really valued and somehow made me feel I had a hand through Sure Start to improve lives.

Whilst carnival offers a chance to 'break the rules' and challenge social norms, at the same time it aspires to join 'civilised' society, resulting in a struggle of 'complex dialectical duality' (Riggio 2004b, p. 44). Thus, as well as idealising the 'outlaw who has the nerve to break the rules', the motivating impulse is also to obtain respectability [since] very few vagabonds treasure their poverty or their pariah status; mostly, they want to be respectable, to be enfranchised, to have a stake in the system they take so much pleasure in metaphorically (and sometimes literally) mooning.

(ibid.)

There was certainly a sense, at this stage of the project, of those involved in the research wanting to be taken seriously and to impress authority figures. Sure Start mothers were pleased with the level of positive response, and especially the emotional reaction that the work elicited:

Cos I wouldn't have expected – well I didn't expect – you know like for't have people being touched by it, moved by it, and you know being able to like relate to it. I remember my social worker. She was in tears. Which was nice, you know, for her to be proud of like what we did and that.

The women involved in the research reported having enjoyed the arts-based groups because, despite the fact that all of the work involved them telling their own stories, paradoxically it felt far removed from their day-to-day lives. Laughter was ever present, particularly in the drama group as participants struggled to learn lines and dance routines. Getting dressed up in ridiculous costumes can also be seen to offer an escape from reality. Other groups on offer at the Sure Start programme were much more instructive and instrumental (such as IT training and parenting classes), resulting in a certificate and fulfilling the Sure Start objective of enhancing job opportunities for out-of-work mothers. In comparison, the drama, art, film-making and poetry seemed an almost frivolous way of spending our time. As Terry Eagleton (2004, p. 39) observes, 'sheer pointlessness is a deeply subversive affair', and the notion of 'doing something purely for the delight of it has always rattled the grey-bearded guardians of the state'. In this age of high capitalism, 'anything which is not useful, which has no immediate cash-value, is a form of sinful self-indulgence' (ibid., p. 86).

Yet in my applications for funding, initially for the art group and later for the research project, I made claims, not necessarily for 'immediate cash-value', but certainly for a longer term investment through 'capacity building'. I highlighted the positive impact on participants' well-being and also strategically employed the concepts of 'social capital' and 'cultural capital' to stress the benefits of our activities. I am not wholly comfortable with this terminology. Ruth Levitas (2004, p. 50) understands how it seems to 'reinforce the normalization and naturalization of capitalism itself, and thus to be part of a discourse which constructs "there is no alternative" without even having to say it'. She continues:

To value, or even describe the skills, attributes, and developed capacities of a person or persons as 'human capital' is to treat those persons as means to an end, in this case capitalist production, rather than as ends in themselves ... Similarly 'social capital' treats the human interactions and solidarities of daily life that are currently outside the market as investment with implied later pay-off, rather than the stuff of life itself.

(ibid.)

Whilst, on one hand, the research project being solely about 'the stuff of life' was appealing, on the other, there was certainly an educative element to the project. These two elements are not necessarily in opposition; education can, and should, be life-enhancing. However, the notion of education in the current climate tends to be highly instrumental and all about securing gainful employment. All of us involved, including me, acquired a lot of new skills as well as knowledge about ourselves and others. I initially set up a basic skills group for community researchers to access in order to develop their reading and writing skills. This continued to develop outside of the research project, and at Sure Start parents' request the tutor went on to offer mathematics classes as well. One of the community researchers that I had initially recruited actually left the research project because she gained the qualifications through the basic skills groups to begin a full-time college course, 'And if I hadn't done that [basic skills] course there's no way I'd have [been able to do it] – 'cause it refreshes you, reminds you'.

The community researchers who did see the project through accompanied me to various academic conferences to co-present the findings of the research. None of them had been inside a university before and they were initially nervous. The papers we gave (supplemented with visual images and film footage) were very well received. At one conference, however, there was an over-enthusiastic response to our paper. We received a thunderous round of applause compared with the polite ripple that other presenters were met with. Whilst some members of our group were delighted with this response, others felt patronised. One Sure Start mother said that she felt like my 'performing monkey'. This experience recalled the art group trips from several years earlier, and I recognised the irony of me trying to imbue the women with middle-class norms and values through educative experiences, when this was something the project championed against. The further I have progressed in my academic career, the more effort it takes to resist being 'ideologically impregnated' (Carey 2011, p. 231) through my role and status. Kathleen Lynch (2000, p. 74) poses the question of whether the academy, 'which is so deeply implicated in the cultural reproduction of elites' can indeed 'facilitate emancipatory change *via* research and education'. Back to the carnival, and Neil Ravenscroft and Paul Gilchrist (2009, p. 36) argue that it is also capable of maintaining the status quo. Carnivalesque inversions of the everyday 'can be, and are, deployed to maintain and reinforce social order and, thus, the discipline of bodies and behaviours'. These inversions are temporary and provide a means of 'allowing ordinary people to feel that they have some freedoms and that they are valued members of the community' (ibid., p. 40).

Conclusion

This chapter has suggested that the participatory arts-based research project at the Sure Start programme can be understood as carnivalesque. The community is 'allied with artistic expression' (Riggio 2004a, p. 20) during a liminal period where social hierarchies are reversed and future outcomes are uncertain. The Sure Start women took charge, resisted convention and presented a colourful alternative to hegemonic representations of poor working-class mothers. However, the extent to which any lasting changes can be made is questionable. The carnivalesque is replete with paradoxes and these mirror issues that arise in the endeavour to undertake an emancipatory approach to knowledge production. As earlier chapters of the book have argued, there are no easy answers to these conundrums. Quaylan Allen's (2012) visual research (discussed in Chapter 4) successfully enabled young Black men to communicate aspects of their lives to a wide audience, including their teachers. However, these aspects of their lives were ones which remained relatively faithful to the standard 'script' that young Black men tend to follow (and its preoccupation with playing sports and flirting with the opposite sex). The work carried out by older people in Trish Hafford-Letchfield et al.'s (2010) research project 'RUDE (Rude Old People)' (discussed in Chapter 5) confronted spectators with the message that older women can enjoy an active sex life, but the participants themselves felt that the project 'never went far enough' – bypassing such taboo topics as masturbation (p. 614) – thus failing to address their younger audience with as much force as they would have liked. The Sure Start research encountered similar dilemmas not only in its tendency to tell the stories that would appeal to certain audiences, but also in the reactions from these various audiences (the over-enthusiastic academics, for instance, and the Sure Start workers keen for their share of the glory).

Despite the uncertainty around the ability of such projects to make the desired change (whether this is desired by researchers or participants or both), there remain myriad possibilities for creating new knowledge through a collaborative arts-based methodology and for pleasure to be had through the process. Hafford-Letchfield et al. (2010) for instance describe the laughter that was a substantive aspect of their research process, and report comments from the older participants on the project such as: 'Loved it, thoroughly enjoyed it all' (p. 612). Two years after the Sure Start research project ended I was awarded further funding from the ESRC which enabled me to revisit the Sure Start community and reflect on the 'lasting legacy' of the research.[2] A series of in-depth interviews took place with the community researchers whose over-riding memories of this period was that it had been 'fun'. We had forged friendships, explored new avenues and, above all, as one Sure Start mother recalls, 'We had a laugh, didn't we?'

The use of humour certainly played a pivotal role throughout the project. Tyler (2008, p. 23) discusses how the lower classes are frequently ridiculed. Laughter is boundary forming and creates distance between 'them' and 'us', asserting moral judgements and a superior class position. Here, however, this was subverted, and it was the Sure Start staff that were gently derided and made fun of. The parents also laughed at themselves through the parody that is 'organically inherent' in carnivalised genres (Bakhtin 1984, p. 128). Parents exaggerated their 'grotesque bodies' with fanciful costumes in the pantomime and *Wizard of Us* play. They exaggerated their 'deviance' in the short film, through bad language and rule-breaking. Bakhtin (1968/1984, p. 89), in his study of Rabelais and medieval folk culture, writes extensively about the subversive power of laughter, discussing its 'indissoluble and essential relation to freedom'. It is life affirming, healing and politically progressive.

Revisiting the community, the progressive nature of the project's impact was, however, questionable. It soon became evident that the divide between staff and parents, particularly those parents who volunteered at the Sure Start programme, had, if anything, increased. Despite the research findings emphatically presenting the Sure Start mothers as 'real mums', they were no longer allowed access to the staff kitchen.

Whilst the emotional responses that the dissemination of research findings elicited suggest an empathic response to the Sure Start mothers (which was one of the objectives of employing arts-based methods in the research), this can be problematic if it is a 'passive' response and does not result in positive change (Boler 1997). Carnivalisations may enable an audience to see the world from the protagonists' perspective, but it is the receptiveness of that audience that decides how effective the process is at challenging social norms.

Yet, despite these organisational limits, there were positive, life-enhancing changes that came from our involvement in the research project. These were no doubt in part due to the educational aspects of the project, such as the skills that were acquired as well as the confidence gained. Every bit as importantly, though, was our 'opening up' to one another and sharing our lives and experiences in a supportive environment. This all contributed to a series of individual and shared achievements. For instance, on my return to the Sure Start community, one of the women who had worked as a community researcher had embarked on a teaching degree at a local university (which she has subsequently graduated from with first class honours). Another had actually secured paid employment with the Sure Start programme which, whilst certainly improving the quality of her life through the gaining of a more secure financial position, rather evokes Millie Taylor's (2007, p. 18) description of the stories of pantomime:

> [T]here is disruption of the accepted order as the young hero alters his status through wit, wisdom and courage, but the resolution restores the status quo, albeit with a hero in a new place within the hierarchy. This can be seen as optimistic in allowing that there is opportunity for transformation and change, or pessimistic in the confrontation of the class-based materialistic society.

The drama group, art group and creative writing group continued to run for some time after our research project had come to an end. When they did stop running, some of the families that had been involved kept up with their new interests. One of the community researchers had particularly enjoyed writing poetry and had gone on to win a competition, through which she had an opportunity to read some of her work on local radio and to have it displayed on public transport. Another mother had thoroughly enjoyed working on the pantomime, along with her children. She had gone on to join a local gospel choir and her daughters were having dance lessons. At the time of writing, I take great pleasure in seeing the family each Christmas at the local pantomime, and last year the girls were dancing in it for the first time.

The carnivalesque tells us that 'the nature of social reality is malleable', as is our place within it (Martin and Renegar 2007, p. 310). Through co-ordinating 'the post-Enlightenment notion of social improvement with the medieval one of community', we are, says Prentki (2009b, p. 367) 'always walking on the edge of possibility'. Whilst the carnival may have come to an end, its spirit can live on in very real ways as we go about our lives. Chapter 7 draws on this idea in its attempt to reframe thinking about the successes and failures of collaborative arts-based research for social justice. It is perhaps the less tangible elements of research projects that hold the most potential for 'doing good'.

Notes

1   ESRC CASE award, 2003–2006. Grant reference: PTA-033-2003-00024.
2   ESRC postdoctoral fellowship, 2008–2009. Grant reference: PTA-026-27-1870.

7 'What is it good for?'

Evaluating the quality, beauty and 'impacts' of arts-based research

Words of self-construction

You're not my architect.
No matter how much you try to draw my plans, your technical knowledge,
intricate designs, use qualifications to undermine,
I'm under construction.
Progress in development.
Not a development opportunity for you to seize without consent
Using my keys, attempting to impose my interior
You're inferior

(Nadine Bourne [Video 14])

Evaluating the successes and failures of research that employs collaborative arts-based methodology in order to promote social justice is no straightforward process. Previous chapters have provided plentiful examples of projects that have employed this methodology with outcomes that are not clear-cut. For instance, research employing poetry as a means of dissemination (such as Finley's [2000] *Dream Child* discussed in Chapter 4) is often triumphant in capturing emotion, yet it cannot speak for everyone. However imaginative and compelling the work may be, it has limits in terms of whose voice dominates, and any claims to truth need to be tempered with this. Jennifer Eisenhauer's (2012) digital stories created by people diagnosed with psychiatric disabilities pose a fitting challenge to the stigmatising depictions of mental health issues in society (discussed in Chapter 3). However, persuading an audience to *hear* these voices and take on board the difficult and uncompromising messages of the research is no effortless task. My Sure Start research discussed in the previous chapter led to a series of worthwhile *individual* transformations, but faltered when it came to producing organisational change.

There may be limitations to these projects, but there is also much scope for posing challenges to the status quo and working together with marginalised groups in ways that promote compassion and lift people's spirits. To this end, this chapter argues that there needs to be much more imaginative thinking around what arts-based research can accomplish. Traditional positivist and post-positivist criteria of validity and reliability, rigour and value-neutrality make little sense when applied to the creative inquiry that is the focus of this book. These are research endeavours that are consciously political, that wilfully abandon claims to objectivity and that play spiritedly with ideas of truth and fiction. To apply exacting criteria of judgement in such a context can be limiting and constraining. Research that is understood as 'messy' and paradoxical, complex and partial, that constructs 'a stuttering knowledge' and 'elicits an experience of the object through its very failures of representation' (Lather 2010, p. 137), cannot be so easily pinned down. Rather it refuses 'assumptions of truth as an adequation of thought to its object and language as a transparent medium of reflection' (ibid., p. 136). The sorts of representations that are produced through arts-based research are 'capable of conveying a sense of truth, but simultaneously undermining its grounds'; these are 'not declarations of what is the case, so much as invitations to "consider this way of seeing the world"' (Gergen and Gergen 2010, para. 9).

Moreover, this is inquiry that gives weight to the experiences and understandings of marginalised people, the intimacies and routines of their everyday lives, and as such is at risk of being automatically consigned to an inferior status (particularly in the academy, but also further afield). Of course, the ultimate goal of social justice-oriented research might be to democratise ways of knowing and to iron out these differences in status (Humphries 2008, p. 194). However, the fact remains that knowledge production is a powerful way of maintaining the oppressive status quo, of transmitting ideology. The search for a master narrative or single truth has reduced the language of analysis to 'white, hegemonic forms of clarity' (McLaren, cited in Ledwith and Springett 2010, p. 125) and it proves difficult to challenge this epistemic violence. Yet it remains as important as ever to attempt to do so. Through the very process of recognising and questioning whose criteria and standards are being used to judge knowledge production, possibilities for positive change emerge. There are a number of tactics that may be employed to this end. The notion of 'nonmastery', for instance, might provide an 'ethical move' (Lather 2010, p. 146). It is in its willingness to expose vulnerability and embrace ambiguity that collaborative arts-based research holds power to make positive changes in people's lives. Artistic transformation is driven by '[u]ncertainty and mystery rather than reliability and predictability' (McNiff 1998, p. 43).

The acknowledgement of the emotional decisions involved in producing and evaluating knowledge is another way of taking a stand against normative strictures. There is little written about emotion in the context of judging the quality and validity of research, but as an antidote to rational discourses it is crucial. As has been argued in previous chapters, one of the main strengths of arts-based research is its affective dimension and its capacity to move participants and viewers into action. There is an undercurrent of anger to this chapter, an appropriate emotion for 'matters connected to social justice' (Snowber and Bickel 2015, p. 73). Anger has the ability to energise its subjects and to move them into 'a different bodily world' (Ahmed 2004, p. 175):

> If anger pricks our skin, if it makes us shudder, sweat and tremble, then it might just shudder us into new ways of being; it might just enable us to inhabit a different kind of skin, even if that skin remains marked or scarred by that which we are against.

Because the arts offer an ideal conduit for emotion, they have the potential to reach a wide audience in potentially affecting ways. However, the stories told through arts-based research accounts are likely to draw a different audience from those told through scholarly or scientific means. These distinct approaches to communicating knowledge can be further differentiated in terms of their 'power and ability to travel and exert influence in the world' (Lyons 2008, p. 81). Not least due to issues of status, the audience for the knowledge produced through collaborative arts-based research is likely to lie outside the domain of the academy and policy makers (although this is not inevitable). Resultant changes might therefore be small-scale, but this does not mean that they are unimportant. Yet to make *any* changes, to have *any* influence, research needs to effectively stir an audience. Dani Snyder-Young opines that no matter which aesthetic forms are used to present data, 'quality matters'; if it is just 'plain old *bad*, it achieves few of its goals to democratize scholarship and engage broader audiences' (2010, p. 891; italics in the original). In terms of furthering social justice then, there is a need to have some notion of the quality of arts-based methods that are employed to disseminate research findings. Many projects will also have to account for the success (or otherwise) of their research outcomes to funding bodies or community organisations. So here as well there is a need for some justification for the approach taken and the resultant work. Yet there are ways of doing this that do not mean accepting oppressive constraints. Criteria are not found; they are made (Bochner 2000, p. 269). It is time to think about making 'new and more ambiguous criteria' (Gergen and Gergen 2010, para. 12).

Once again a tightrope-walk is necessary, this time between prescriptive evaluative criteria and an 'anything goes' attitude. What is most important to heed is that there is nothing neutral about this balancing act; it is a moral and an ethical practice (Denzin and Giardina 2010, p. 12). In order to strike a balance, Patti Lather (2010, p. 119) argues for a new counter-discourse or practice of legitimation. Without this we are bound to 'revert to the dominant foundational, formulaic, and readily available codes of validity'. These are dangerous. A politics or system that does not leave space for alternative realities is 'the enactment of its own exquisite form of cruelty' (Law 2004, p. 97). The first section in this chapter, 'A new fable', provides an example of the violence that dominant epistemology can perform. Employing strict evaluative criteria extends this violence. There are suggestions made as to what a counter-discourse might look like, but without being prescriptive and replacing one set of rules with another. The section 'Challenging criteria' extends this discussion and gives consideration to alternative notions of 'generalisability' and 'validity'. These are criteria that need to be flexible enough to be able to be 'fitted to the pragmatic, ethical and political contingencies of concrete situations' (Denzin and Lincoln 2011, p. 564).

Criteria for evaluating qualitative work require a blending of ethics and epistemologies, and also of *aesthetics* (Denzin and Lincoln 2002, p. 229). Aesthetics (theories of beauty) play a role in both art and science in terms of the choices made which go beyond straightforward reason (Sandelowski 1994, p. 54). However, they are particularly pronounced in arts-based approaches to knowledge production. The section 'Aesthetic battles: round one', then, considers the 'quality' of the products of arts-based research and the skill needed to produce them. It argues that there is a need to move beyond traditional Western understandings of aesthetics, which can be elitist and limiting, in order to consider the ways that aesthetics can contribute to furthering social justice. 'Aesthetics battles: round two' continues this discussion in relation to the 'utility' of the arts. For instance, Maggie O'Neill et al. (2002, p. 78) describe art works as 'ciphers of the social world' and a means of accessing 'the "sedimented stuff" of society – what is normally unseen/hidden/ overlooked'. The function of aesthetics is thus 'to reveal the unintentional truths about the social. Arts-based research methods therefore require not only a re-evaluation of truth and knowledge, but also of beauty' (Leavy 2009, p. 17).

This discussion is followed by 'Resisting commodification', which considers the ways that collaborative arts-based research might address issues of consumption and possession in relation to its research outputs. Such an issue is particularly pertinent in the academy, not least in terms of what counts as knowledge and the increasing expectation on academics to fit into a particular mould. Finding ways around this involves building new relationships on an individual as well as a collective scale. The section 'Being kind' elaborates on the potential for these interactions to make positive changes. It argues that in order to achieve a research model grounded in 'concepts of care, shared governance, neighbourliness, love and kindness' (Denzin and Lincoln 2002, p. 229) these qualities need to be enacted on a daily basis.

A new fable

Linda Tuhiwai Smith's (2012) account of the way that the West has taken ownership of indigenous people's worlds, systematically denying the validity of indigenous people's knowledge, bristles with anger. How can it not when this has resulted in communities living in abject poverty and at risk of having their children forcibly removed from their care (ibid., p. 4)? The Western tradition of rationality has meant that scientific accounts have been judged as superior to 'primitive' accounts of indigenous people (ibid., p. 172), despite the atrocities that they have wrought. The disservice of research is not deliberate. Researchers for the most part see their work as contributing to the greater good and assume that they are representatives of such an ideal (ibid., p. 2). Yet the reality is that, without a very considered attempt to counter this, the outcome of research is a direct reflection of the dominant ideology. One way of posing a challenge to the status quo is to acknowledge that indigenous people have valuable 'counter-stories' to tell. These can powerfully resist the authorising knowing of imperial and colonial practices.

Smith (2012, pp. 174–175) describes the importance of knowledge in traditional Maori society, and tells the tale of how knowledge was first gained, a startlingly different story from Western accounts. It was Tane-nui-a-rangi, a child of the first woman (formed from a mound of earth) and the male sky spirit, who made a journey to the twelfth 'universe' to seek knowledge on behalf of the community. This knowledge was separated into three baskets, each containing a particular, specialised knowledge that was regarded as essential to collective well-being and survival. Although there was a hierarchy in terms of who was entrusted with this knowledge, there was also a requirement that those with specialist knowledge or skills held them on behalf of others. They would simultaneously be dependent on others who held other vital skills. Members of the group were thus interdependent in quite complex ways.

Jo-Ann Archibald (2008, p. 2), in her work on indigenous stories, continues to employ the basket as a metaphor for gaining knowledge, in this case for learning about storytelling. She refers to the complex designs of Stó:lō and Coast Salish baskets, designs that whilst they may be particular to one person, reflect relationships with 'family, community, nation, land, and nature'. Teachings that are communicated through stories are about 'respect, reverence, responsibility, holism, interrelatedness and synergy'. It follows then, as Smith (2012, p. 176) argues, that if an outside researcher to the indigenous community is to question individual informants (as is often the case), there is going to be much missing from the complex network of interwoven knowledge, experience and history. However much vigilance is taken to select an appropriate research methodology and to ensure analytical rigour, reliability and validity, there is not going to be a sense of the whole picture; carefully fashioned patterns will be distorted. It is not a matter 'of looking harder or more closely, but of seeing what frames our seeing – spaces of constructed visibility and incitements to see which constitute power/ knowledge' (Lather 2010, p. 119).

Dwight Conquergood (2002, p. 146) drolly observes that in the academy there is 'no contest' between methodologically 'rigorous', objective knowledge and local, community-based knowing; it is 'the choice between science and old wives' tales'. Yet there is increasing acknowledgement that the ubiquitous evidence-based approach to generating and evaluating knowledge is itself a 'fable' (Denzin and Giardina 2010, p. 30). A new fable is necessary, and there are certain elements that this fable might be constructed around. These include an acknowledgement that 'objectivity' and 'evidence' are political and ethical terms, and that inquiry is always political and moral. Empirical materials should be understood as performative as opposed to commodities for our consumption. There is also an emphasis on 'openness'. So although there may be a need for an 'ample supply' of methodological rules and guidelines, these are open to interpretation, reflecting that inquiry is 'open-ended, unruly, disruptive' (ibid.). The notion of a single 'gold standard' is to be abhorred and there is a need to keep methodology 'open, alive, loose' (Lather 2010, p. x). Spiritual teacher Mooji (Video 15) advises:

When you define yourself you confine yourself also … Every word seems to have some limitation. Use all the words, use any concept at all, but don't lock them, leave some space open, leave some space. Then you can use any concept, you don't have to tie them around your neck … you don't have to make tattoos out of any teaching, just use them, see what they're pointing to.

This focus on openness, ambiguity and error is at odds with more conventional approaches to research. Their inclination tends toward 'achieving a kind of closure', a desire that is bound up with 'reducing uncertainty about the truthfulness and usefulness of knowledge claims' (Barone 2001, p. 24). If research is going to move forwards from this static, shuttered-up position (a position which keeps knowledge safely held within the domain of the powerful), an epistemological humility is required. The German aesthetic concept of *freischwebend* is useful in this regard. Meaning, literally, 'to hover above', it suggests that 'not everything is knowable'; there requires an acceptance that: 'Knowing requires not knowing: a state of being lost in order to find' (Siegesmund and Cahmann-Taylor 2008, p. 234).

Challenging criteria

Any criteria that are employed in evaluating arts-based research need to reflect this uncertainty and ambiguity. This requires a particular state of mind, 'a fluid stream rather than a fixed rock' (Eisner 2008b, p. 25). Engaging reflectively with the arts can enable the development of this state of mind, this 'wisdom'. It is wisdom that 'distinguishes between what we can positively affect and what is beyond our grasp' (Siegesmund and Cahmann-Taylor 2008, p. 234). And it is this same wisdom that can enable us to make connections between the particular and the general, 'between the instance and aspects of the world that were not initially part of that instance' (Eisner 2008b, p. 21). As this ability to see connections is sharpened, an alternative notion to that of the traditional research concept of 'generalisability' is produced. In arts-based research there are no random samples, no comparable sets of conditions or statistical generalisations to be made. Rather, samples are likely to be small and replete with their own peculiarities. It is the development of a questioning, reflective mind that 'will enable us to peer more deeply into situations that might not be the same as the ones we study' (ibid.).

Arts-based inquiry draws attention to the intricate processes of daily life; their idiosyncrasies. It is, however, when work and life 'crash into each other in a head on collision' that 'the most charged intellectual insights occur' (Behar 2008, p. 63). Poetic anthropologist Ruth Behar discusses the wrenching example of when she was researching attitudes towards death in Spain. At the same time, back in America, her beloved grandfather died. Making painful connections between the research and her personal loss, Behar (after some time) was able to honour both through an insightful piece of writing that brought them together, 'though in real life they were completely separate' (indeed they were separated by entire continents). Behar provides a second example of making connections between different worlds in order to create a new, deeper understanding. She carried out dialogic research in Mexico with a survivor of child abuse and domestic abuse, an 'aggressive, self-assured' single mother and street peddler of Indian heritage who, Behar acknowledges, could not be more different from her. Yet through exploring the conjunctures of their lives, stories resulted that took on a force of their own. They have been read widely by Latino and Latina students 'trying to understand the lives of their Latin American mothers', as well as by women in prison 'interrogating the violence in their lives' (ibid., p. 64).

Not only does this suggest that evocative accounts of the particular have the scope to travel, it also begins to address the notion of validity. In qualitative research, validity refers to the way that a study 'convinces others of its soundness or quality' (Freeman 2011, p. 544). Patti Lather (2010, p. 118) ponders on the obsession (her own included) with validity and legitimation issues in research methodology. There is undoubtedly recognition from certain quarters that the traditions we draw on in terms of assessing these mistakes are 'no longer adequate to the task' (ibid., p. 127). Lather plays with a 'transgressive' validity checklist, replete with 'scandalous categories'. These are intended to disrupt standardisation and work against 'the inscription of another "regime of truth"' (ibid., p. 120). The categories include 'ironic' validity, 'paralogical' validity, 'rhizomatic' validity and 'voluptuous' validity.

In brief summary, ironic validity gives weight to the insufficiency of language, problems of representation and the 'problem' of truth. 'Paralogical' refers to Lyotardian theory with its goal of fostering differences, acknowledging complexities and allowing contradictions to remain in tension with one another. Rhizomatic validity derives from Derridean rigour. Like a rhizome spreading underground and sending out unsettling roots and shoots on its way, it works against 'constraints of authority via relay, multiple openings, networks, complexities of problematics'. Voluptuousness brings in the 'disruptive excess' of the female imaginary and contrasts it with the phallocentric position that attempts to divide ethics from epistemology. Voluptuous validity highlights risky, explicit yet partial knowledge and situated practice.

All of these categories – the final one in particular – highlight the need to transcend the rational and to embrace multifarious mysteries and paradox. There remains a requirement for researchers using arts-based data to be 'in tune to their emotional, carnal, psychological, and intellectual indicators' (Leavy 2009, p. 48). This is no place for the disavowal of feelings, as researchers have traditionally been taught. Rather, these 'internal signals are vital to building authentic and trustworthy knowledge' (ibid., p. 49). Peter Willis employs the concept of 'verisimilitude' in this context and describes this as a '"phenomenological aha" – the moment of "that's it"; "yes that is what it's really like"' (2008, p. 54). This is not dissimilar to the notion of 'aesthetic resonance', which similarly involves recognition of research 'accuracy' through a trust in sensory mechanisms (Richardson 1990b, p. 17). Art Bochner (2000, p. 270), in the context of evaluating alternative ethnography, describes how he ascertains whether or not a story is 'good'. Among other factors, it needs to include 'abundant concrete details' of people's everyday lives and their emotional response to coping with these. It might also capture 'contradictory feelings, ambivalence, and layers of subjectivity, squeezing comedy out of life's tragedies'. Finally, he says,

> I want a story that moves me, my heart and belly as well as my head; I want a story that doesn't just refer to subjective life, but instead acts it out in ways that show me what life feels like now and what it can mean.

> (ibid.)

It is in this sense that intuition and the imagination can be understood as important factors in being able to recognise 'truths' constructed through the research process, and it would be imprudent to neglect such a creative and embodied response when judging the authenticity of research.

In terms of furthering social justice, Terry Jenoure (2008, p. 175) evaluates the success of her arts-based research by considering 'how fruitful' it has been: whether it has inspired and motivated; whether it has opened doors to 'unexplored frontiers'. This does not necessarily mean that the research has successfully met its aims. For instance, as Josh Packard's (2008) account of research with homeless men (discussed in Chapter 4) demonstrates, even when the outcomes of research are not 'successful', their very failings hold important lessons and raise fruitful questions in terms of social inequality and injustice. Patti Lather (2010, p. 148) raises similar conclusions in respect of her 'Angels' project (discussed in Chapter 3) which worked with women with HIV/AIDS: 'perhaps it is the very questioning engagement of our intervention that is the politics of what we have done'.

Aesthetic battles: round one

Whilst all research has to contend with notions of insufficiency and inadequacy, these are often highlighted in arts-based research. Included in the list of offences that David Pariser (2009, p. 9) levels at arts-based research is that it is 'neither good research nor good art'. This concept of quality of both the knowledge and the art work that emerges from the process is important to consider especially if, as discussed above, the desire is to affect positive social change and to be taken seriously by funders and organisations, if not the academy. Melisa Cahnmann-Taylor (2008, p. 11) understands that arts-based research is at risk of '"anything goes" criteria, making it impossible to distinguish what is excellent from what is amateur'. She stresses the need to build a critical community of arts-based researchers, and this requires both training in arts-based methods and a sharing among researchers of 'techniques and aesthetic sensibilities'. This focus on application is important because, as Cahnmann-Taylor observes, there is more work describing arts-based research criteria than there is about examples of the work itself.

Susan Finley (2008, p. 72) discusses the tension that exists in arts-based research between 'artistic excellence' and 'political effectiveness'. She notes that a researcher's criteria for excellence 'do not always harmonise' with those held by artists for a particular form. In this regard, the products of research practice perhaps need to be understood as 'arts-*based*' rather than 'fully-fledged art' (Barone 2001, p. 25; italics in the original). Monica Prendergast (2009, pp. xxv–xxvi), however, describes this position as being 'on the safer side of the fence'. She notes that Corrine Glesne (1997) takes a similar position in terms of the use of the poetic in research. This 'moves in the direction of poetry but is not necessarily poetry' (cited in Prendergast 2009, p. xxv). Others are more inclined to think that arts-based researchers should have some aesthetic qualifications. Jane Piirto (2002, p. 443) sways toward this view given the 'painful' act of observing 'heartfelt efforts' by researchers who had no background in the art form they were using. This was amplified if audience members were trained in that art. Whilst social scientists' training would certainly be greatly enriched through adding in arts and creative writing training (indeed this is something that, at the time of writing, I am starting to include in research methods courses for both undergraduate and postgraduate students), this is currently the exception rather than the norm. I would also argue that it is not a necessity in terms of adopting a collaborative arts-based approach. As examples through the book have demonstrated, successful collaborations can be made with artists and performers that remove this pressure on researchers. Moreover, researchers are frequently capable of producing engaging, thought-provoking and aesthetically appealing work themselves without formal training in the arts, such as Susan Finley's (2000) or Deborah Austin's (1996) poetry, or Moshoula Capous-Desylla's (2015) art work (see Chapter 4 for discussion of these examples). It is, however, researched communities who are often involved in the production of artistic data when adopting this methodological approach, and this adds a further layer to discussions of what constitutes quality.

Research participants themselves are frequently concerned over whether their work is 'good enough'. Darlene Clover (2007, p. 92) discusses how many adults have 'a very impoverished sense of their own creative possibilities'. She describes the 'challenge or risk' in learning that comes from learning to be creative. Of course, this also means that arts-based methods can be excluding if potential participants do not have the confidence to attempt them. For instance, one of the findings from my research at the Sure Start programme described the painful lack of confidence and self-esteem that so many poor working-class mothers experienced. It often required gentle coaxing to invite them to take part in the arts-based research and undoubtedly it did exclude those who felt unable to do so. Pushed to take these risks, however, participants become 'not only the researched, the researchers, and the knowers, but also, artists' (Clover 2007, p. 92).

Romanie van Son (2000, p. 230) worked with a group of women to explore issues of import to them using a range of visual art techniques. She observed that 'some fluency in visual language needed to be learned during the initial stages of the project'. Allowing 'space and freedom to play was very important, particularly to women who only began to get really involved once they realised they could do "their own thing" and that "perfect results" didn't matter' (ibid., p. 222). The results, captured and re-produced by van Son through colour photographs, are startling. An array of methods, from clay and wirework models, through to painting have been utilised and the range of work produced is reminiscent of 'outsider art'. Interestingly, Colin Rhodes (2000, p. 20), writing about this genre of art that is produced outside the mainstream of contemporary Western art, observes that, for living outsider artists, problems relating to quality only arise when the work begins to garner a national and international audience. The work's status 'only becomes problematical at the point at which they begin to move "inside"'.

Darlene Clover and Joyce Stalker (2007, pp. 12–13), writing in the context of employing the arts in adult education in order to further social justice, outline the tensions between process and finished product in terms of promoting learning and social justice. They argue that if art works are produced for personal and/or therapeutic reasons then the issue of quality is not necessarily relevant. However, if the work does aim to engage the public in terms of educating and enlightening, then quality is often 'key to its impact' (ibid.). Clover, in quilting projects with young women exploring sexual exploitation (discussed in Chapter 3) and in other projects involving social justice-oriented quilts that aimed to 'provoke aesthetic oppositional messages', came to realise the value of quality when the final pieces were displayed at a traditional quilt show (2007, p. 95). The quilts were examined by quilters from around the world who were initially hesitant about the confrontational subject matter. However, as they came to recognise the quality of the craftwork involved, they also began to engage with the ideas expressed. Engendering an aesthetic experience in viewers or readers is a way of making connections, establishing empathy, touching emotions, disturbing equilibrium and rendering the status quo questionable. They can encourage dialogue in which 'ideas and ideals may be shared for the purposes of an improved reality. Plots may be hatched against inadequate present conditions in favour of more emancipatory social arrangements in the future' (Barone 2008, p. 39).

Aesthetic battles: round two

Judging the quality of stitchwork is perhaps less subjective than judging the quality of painting or a story. This has links with the fact that there is very much a hierarchy of arts from the 'low' world of craft to the 'high' world of fine art (see Auther 2009 for example). There is also similar judgement in performing arts, with opera and ballet, for example, drawing very different audiences from the more lowbrow ones of pantomime such as we performed during the course of the Sure Start research. Aesthetic judgements tend to involve elitist criteria. This stems from the Kantian notion that beauty lies in the judgement made by the person viewing an object rather than in the object itself (Winston 2006, p. 288). These judgements of taste are universalised; they make universal claims to the validity of an aesthetic experience. Winston points out that, following this line of argument, it becomes a duty of education to identify 'good taste' and beauty and to educate young people into it. Thus beauty becomes, to use Bourdieu's term, a form of cultural capital. If only a select few are privy to understandings of good taste and beauty this is 'a form of snobbery and status seeking and a contributory force to social exclusion'. Janet Wolff's work has stressed that works of art are not universal; rather they are shaped by social and historical processes and are not 'above' social divisions and prejudices (Wolff 1993, p. 28). Of course, that does not mean that aesthetics should be devalued. On the contrary, beauty adds much meaning to our lives and because of this it must not be reserved for the privileged few. As Winston (2006, p. 288) points out, beauty remains a commonly used word in people's daily lives, 'within contexts where ordinary people know perfectly well what they are talking about and what they mean'.

Denzin and Lincoln (2002, p. 230) argue that '[a]ll aesthetics and standards of judgement are based on particular moral standpoints'. Drawing on the work of Patricia Hill Collins (1990), they describe an Afrocentric feminist aesthetic. This acknowledges the importance of truth, knowledge and beauty through 'experiential, communal, and shared' wisdom and storytelling. This is wisdom that is 'derived from local, lived, familial and communal experience, and expresses lore, folktale, and myth' (ibid.). Christine Ballengee-Morris's work on indigenous aesthetics similarly highlights traditions and rituals. It also stresses the relationship between individual and collective identities. There is a strong focus in Native art on spirituality and nature; the ways in which nature is expressed through indigenous art 'connects space and spirituality' and ties to the land unite communities (2008, p. 31). This is quite different from Western approaches to aesthetics where the spiritual dimension tends to be overlooked. It therefore makes sense, says Ballengee-Morris, to understand indigenous aesthetics from 'within these notions and not from colonial frameworks' (ibid., p. 32).

In the UK, over recent years, a certain amount of ambivalence can be detected when it comes to assessing the value of the arts. There is a tendency to view them from an instrumentalist agenda (Cowling 2004; Matarasso 1997) and to acknowledge their utility in terms of improving educational standards and encouraging social cohesion (Winston 2006). There is currently much focus on the health benefits of the arts (see Gordon-Nesbitt 2015; RSPH 2013), and the Arts Council England (2014) has published an evidence review of *The Value of Arts and Culture to People and Society*. This review focuses on four areas: the Economy, Health and Wellbeing, Society, and Education. These are unquestionably important areas and being able to demonstrate the impact of the arts on each of them means that funding is likely to be forthcoming. One of the most interesting points in the Arts Council England's report is in reference to an IPSOS MORI (2011) report published by the Arts and Humanities Research Council. This establishes that beauty 'is regarded as a positive experience strongly related to bringing about happiness and wellbeing in individuals' lives and that access to beauty is felt to contribute to overall welfare and a "good society"' (2014, p. 11). It acknowledges that intrinsic responses to arts and culture, such as aesthetic pleasure, can thus 'spill over' to more instrumental impacts.

Beauty *can* thus be understood as a force for good. Following Iris Murdoch, Joe Winston (2006, p. 286) reflects how the 'experience of beauty itself can be seen as educational in an active, moral sense' and that there is no need 'to resort to instrumentalist objectives outside of its domain'. As well as being influenced by Murdoch's thesis on beauty, Winston (2006, p. 295) draws on Elaine Scarry's 'elaborate argument' that an education in beauty might be understood as an education in social justice. There is an other-worldliness to beauty: 'Beautiful things always carry greetings from other worlds in them' (Scarry 2001, p. 47, cited in Winston 2006, p. 296). Thus, through engaging the imagination, the viewer is led 'back into her own world with a more capacious regard for it' (Winston 2006, p. 296). Moreover, beauty is dialogic, an interaction between self and other. Beauty enables us to 'gaze with renewed attention and care at those persons or objects within a category we have now recognized as beautiful' (ibid., p. 298). Winston extends this idea to encompass an appreciation for the 'other', including 'disabled' people. Once we are able to appreciate a disabled person for their beauty, 'we extend this acquaintance to others in that category with an innate appreciation of their potential and worth'. With this in mind, I urge readers to watch the performance of Lucy Willer's poem *A Head Like Mine* (Video 16). Lucy was a member of the performance poetry project *Seen but Seldom Heard* outlined in Chapter 5.

A Head Like Mine

It's hard for me with a head like mine
It's difficult trying to talk
People hurry me and don't let me explain
I feel lost and lonely inside my brain

I'm angry, I'm crying, I'm fighting inside
A deadly tiger, I have to hide
If I unleash his teeth and claws and roar
He will tear and bite you all

Talk to me, be patient and calm
Discover the golden monkey that lives in my belly
Release the bird that sings in my heart ...

Lucy's complex disabilities require her to communicate using a communication book. She is thus unable to recite the poem herself. However, she performs the work in the most incredibly beautiful and moving way, articulating her anger with powerful punches and snarls.

The work also illustrates that there are exceptions to any criteria, however sensible it may seem. Darquise Lafrenière and Susan Cox (2013) have devised a meta-framework, an overarching conceptual framework, in order to guide the assessment of the quality and effectiveness of arts-based research (a framework that may well prove useful in terms of their specific aims, which include helping to evaluate scholarly publications and theses, preparing research grants, or designing research projects using arts-based methodologies [ibid., p. 319]). For instance, they assert that in order for an arts-based work to:

> create the desired effects, the performers and environment – facilities and equipment – must be conducive to it. For instance, if a poem or song lyrics are to be read aloud or sung, the individual who will recite or sing must be competent for the task (e.g. demonstrate good diction, intonation, rhythm, etc.).
>
> (ibid., p. 323)

Yet following this criteria would disregard Lucy's performance; a performance of great beauty that offers potential to make the world a better, kinder place. This is in line with Yasmin Gunaratnam's (2009, p. 26) suggestion that 'the value of aesthetic experience ... can be less about the representational qualities of a medium and is more about the mutual social, emotional and corporeal vulnerability that connects us to one another'. Such a vulnerability 'is all too often resisted, denied or avoided in research and in professional practice' (ibid.).

Resisting commodification

In a world driven by the global market, the necessity of reaching out to one another and acknowledging our vulnerability is amplified. In much conventional research, the entire process of fieldwork can involve 'intruding into people's lives, taking their memories, their wisdom and their understanding and making it one's own property' (Fernandes 2003, p. 80). 'Data are commodities', state Denzin and Giardina (2010, p. 20). Produced by researchers, they are frequently owned by the government or by funding agencies. Linda Tuhiwai Smith (2012, p. 93) describes the commercial nature of knowledge 'transfer' in the context of researching the 'Other'. No matter how knowledge is collected or represented, 'people and their culture, the material and the spiritual, the exotic and the fantastic, become not just the stuff of dreams and imagination, or stereotypes and eroticism, but of the first truly global commercial enterprise: *trading the Other*'. This process 'deeply, intimately, defines Western thinking and identity' (ibid.).

Evaluating the success of arts-based research for social justice needs to acknowledge and reflect on the extent to which the work is implicated in this critical issue of commodification. Again, creative thinking is required because when 'conventional, purely visible and material, measures are used as a means of assessment, this often leads to a miscalculation of successes and failures' (Fernandes 2003, p. 120). Of course, it is not just knowledge production that is at risk of commodification. In today's Western societies 'all human experiences (life, eroticism, happiness, recognition)' are tied to commodities, or rather their 'consumption and possession' (Lehmann 2006, p. 183). One of the most troubling outcomes of this is that 'actual relations with and responses to other people have the potential to become marginalised (Grehan 2009, p. 10). Leela Fernandes (2003, p. 90) discusses how people's lives are increasingly shaped by the media that turn people's suffering 'into a spectacle that we safely consume from a distance'. She argues the vital need for researchers to guard against this 'consumption-oriented approach to suffering', in what she understands as a fundamental ethical issue. This is certainly a risk that arts-based research takes. There is concern over the 'aestheticising of social problems' and the way in which visual methods 'can turn poverty into an object of enjoyment' (O'Neill et al. 2002, p. 79). Yet at the same time, art works do have a critical potential to 'pierce us' and grasp the reality of others.

It is in this sense that a case can be argued for positioning arts-based research as 'a tool of resistance against the politics of neo-conservatism' (Finley 2008, p. 71). In the pursuit of such an agenda, questions about the success of arts-based research need to be focused on its contribution to 'progressive social action'. This is not dissimilar from the goals of participatory art which, rather than supplying the market with commodities, seeks to 'channel art's symbolic capital towards constructive social change' (Bishop 2012, p. 13). It is the focus on action and process that is important here. Enabling people to create art works, to bring them into existence, means that 'they are being active producers and transmitters rather than passive consumers of culture' (West and Stalker 2007, p. 135). The process of producing the art work is arguably as important as the product. Processes are replete with meaning, 'metaphors in their own right' (Clover 2007, p. 94).

Responding to art work also necessitates 'conscious participation' (Greene 2000, p. 125). Aesthetic experiences require 'a going out of energy, an ability to notice what is there to be noticed'. This is complicated by the fact that the world of marketing has also shifted 'from communicating "messages" to consumers to providing "experiences" of new products or brands' (Hughes and Ruding 2009, p. 222). One such example is the Kleenex *Let it Out* campaign which was filmed in several British cities. Members of the public were invited to sit on a blue couch, with a well known actor acting as interviewer, to tell their stories and to 'let out' their emotions. This resulted in tears, laughter and hugs (Video 17). Marc Zander, the UK and Ireland marketing manager, describes the campaign's aim to 'create an emotional affinity between the consumer and Kleenex tissues' (utalkmarketing. com 2007). A 7Up campaign recruited the pioneer of urban knitting to create a knitted double-decker bus, a delightfully colourful affair which brightened up the streets of London and in so doing engaged the general public in an affecting aesthetic experience (Video 18). There is thus a need to temper claims for the radical potential of the imagination when it can be engaged in ways that are less than desirable in terms of promoting social justice.

An important role of the arts-based researcher needs to be a facilitator of reflection and dialogue. The imagination may deal 'in unpredictabilities, in the unexpected', but it still requires reflectiveness on our part 'to acknowledge the existence of these unexpected and unpredictable vistas and perspectives in our experiences' (Greene 2000, p. 125). If researchers can encourage this of participants and audiences, there is potential to help communities 'preserve, create and rewrite culture on dynamic indigenous spaces' (Finley 2008, pp. 73–74). It is a strength of collaborative arts-based work that it often takes place outside the walls of elitist institutions and that the work is relocated to 'the realm of local, personal, everyday places and events'. However, this does not necessarily make for an easy life for academics. Even if they succeed in addressing an audience outside of the university, they will still also have to justify their work within its confines, in an environment that is not necessarily sympathetic to the distribution of authority (Servaes 1996, pp. 23–24). Traditional social science has prided itself on its capacity to accumulate knowledge that advances the discipline (Gergen and Gergen 2010, para. 12), and in academic circles there is no escaping 'what we want to rule in and what we want to rule out' (Pelias in conversation, in Denzin and Giardina 2010, p. 324). In this sense academics can be seen as implicated in 'policing' the acceptable content of their disciplines (for instance, through what is published in peer reviewed academic journals), as well as the acceptable evaluative criteria.

In a performance at the 2009 Smithsonian Folklife Festival (Video 19), Omi Osun Joni L. Jones ruminates on the fact that so few professors in the USA are Black women (about 4 per cent): 'We like to think of these academic institutions as lovely, kind, open-minded, generous spaces where we exchange ideas. Well that has not been my experience!' And it's Omi Jones' own experience that she draws on in her performance poem *To the Editor* about having her first academic essay published.

To the Editor

she said she was my sister
but
sisterhood
is being redefined
without my consent

she pressed my hair
and she weren't even my moma
no comfort of familial straightening
no warm momahands on Saturday night
before Sunday school gotta look good

she pressed out the kinks of me-ness
of slash marks and nouns into verbs
and ump humph umph

she thused and therefored my hair to a
stiff straight flatness
a spit polish shine
Dixie Peach
the overpressed awkwardness
apparent in every word

did she know how hard it was to find this nappy freedom
to close away that straightening comb in the kitchen drawer

after all
there was the thousands of years of silence
after all
there was my daily institutionalisation
after all
there was the phd where i was dissed to death
i hope my edges go back real soon
go back from sweat and living.

she said she was my sister
but
sisterhood
is being redefined
without my consent

(Reproduced with kind permission of the poet.)

There is a need for arts-based researchers in the academy to resist this 'straightening' and conforming to standards that best serve careerist White men. Potential exists to do this through recognising the restraints that the academy imposes and using them as an impetus for something different. For instance, one of these restraints includes 'exposing the personal' (Kip Jones 2006b, p. 74). Dissatisfaction with this state of affairs may lead arts-based researchers to seek other avenues for their work, 'new technologies and modes of presentation'; these experiences can bring us back 'to more traditional outlets such as journals and books with a renewed vision for extending the possibilities of traditional publication' (ibid.). The more collective this venture is, the more the academy may open up to the 'inclusion of multiple traditions' and thus 'become more polyvocal, dialogic and democratic' (Gergen and Gergen 2010, para. 9).

Being kind

Posing challenges to the status quo is a collective venture and working collaboratively is crucial. Doing so focuses attention on the qualities of the participative-relational practices in the work. These are issues of 'interdependence, politics, power and empowerment' that must be addressed at both micro and macro levels (Reason and Bradbury 2001, p. 448), from face-to-face interactions through to situating work in a wider political context. What is particularly important here is that there is 'congruence between qualities of participation which we espouse and the actual work we accomplish'. It is too easy to become entangled in complex dynamics of power and to 'identify with the structures of power we are trying to unravel' (Fernandes 2003, p. 45).

So many participatory research projects, whether they use arts-based methods or not, claim to 'empower' participants without sufficient thought or justification as to why this might be the case. Power is not a commodity and cannot be possessed or distributed so effortlessly (Kothari 2001, p. 141).

This idea also calls into question the discourse of social capital and cultural capital.

As discussed in Chapter 6, such terminology 'normalises' and 'naturalises' capitalism as the very basis of human relating (see Levitas 2004). Research that aims to further social justice needs, then, to challenge – or at the very least acknowledge – the profound inequalities that a capitalist economy produces, veiled as they are by a discourse which stubbornly refuses to concede to their existence. It needs to elevate the status of our sensory experiences and relationships, understanding that we are more than just producers and consumers. As researchers there is a responsibility 'to become people who not only believe in social justice and various other ethical or moral values related to the welfare and betterment of humanity but also people who embody these values in the very fibre of our being' (Allman 2001, p. 169). This is essential in order that we do not act in ways that cause damage, for example through 'gossip, slander, and competitiveness':

> While these may seem like small ethical errors compared to more obvious forms of social exclusion, they in fact mirror the same forms of power that underpin social inequalities based on race, sexuality or class, for they violate an understanding of the interconnectedness between all individuals that is crucial for any lasting kind of transformation.
>
> (Fernandes 2003, p. 55)

Mindful awareness of human relationships is thus an important aspect of research that aims to further social justice. Again this involves an acceptance of emotion in the research process and the fact that this cannot be separated from the process of knowledge production. The 'intellectual cover-up of emotion, intuition, and human relationships in the name of expert or academic knowledge' (Wilkins 1993, p. 94) is damaging, not least in terms of the important insights that will be overlooked. In a critique of service user involvement in research, Sarah Carr (2004, p. 16) notes that the direct experience of service users (in particular those with mental health issues or learning difficulties) may be expressed in ways that are regarded as 'too distressing or disturbing'. Not only can this be threatening for professionals, this 'authentic' knowledge occupies second place to knowledge that can claim status of 'evidence'.

There is a need, then, in order to engage with participants' worlds, for a dialectical relationship of a theory of emotion held in critical tension with reason and rationality (O'Neill et al. 2002, p. 83). Learning about others can teach us about ourselves, 'not for the purpose of verifying or solidifying what that means but to enrich the possibilities of living our lives well' (Freeman 2011, p. 549). Whilst this does not mean that we have to directly share these newly acquired understandings with others, it does require of us 'a different relationship to truth than is traditionally conceived' (ibid.), one rooted in connection, and in trusting emotional and bodily experiences and communication. Accordingly, it also means taking responsibility for our actions and being wide-awake to the ways in which we engage with the world (Fels 2015, p. 114). Some understand this as a spiritual process (Fernandes 2003; Anzaldúa 1987; Lorde 2000). The definition of spirituality here is best expressed by the Dalai Lama (1999, p. 22, cited in Fernandes 2003, p. 53), who relates it to qualities 'such as love and compassion, patience, tolerance, forgiveness, contentment, a sense of responsibility, a sense of harmony'. These qualities have in common a concern for the well-being of others and are crucial to social justice aims.

Emphasising the values associated with rationality, equality, individualism and materialism leaves 'little room for emotions and even less room for soul'. Ronald Hustedde and Betty King attempt to define soul, a difficult task given the ambiguity of the concept. They note that the great wisdom traditions see soul as a mysterious force that 'penetrates the illusion of the external world' (Hustedde and King 2002, p. 340). It is thus more than values and ethics, but it makes itself known when people speak of 'compassion, forgiveness, and understanding, and hope amidst despair'. It is within moments of performative action that the 'unsayable, the unspeakable, the unsaid' dwell (Fels 2015, p. 112). Walsh et al. (2015, p. 1) investigate ways of allowing spiritual practice to be present within arts-based research, of finding 'ways of being present – in the moment – and also open to what is not yet known'. To this end the authors have placed a *Lectico Divina* (a meditation or prayer) between each chapter in the volume as a contemplative space for the reader. These take the form of found poems and photographs. The arts enable the opening of the senses that is required to rest and listen. Poems or images provide an accessible way of 'enabling complex and ambivalent interpretations' yet at the same time do not 'offer up otherness on a plate that can be consumed through empathy or easy/ lazy categorisation' (ibid.). Thus the arts offer the hopeful scenario of 'bringing about new and uncertain ways of encountering difference' (Gunaratnam 2009, p. 22). 'People United', a charitable organisation in the UK that promotes participation in the arts, also proposes that the arts offer an opportunity to inspire kindness. This might be through the emotions that they can raise and the connections that they can forge. Or kindness might be encouraged through the opportunities for learning that the arts provide and through an exploration of the human values they address (Broadwood et al. 2012, p. 14).

Conclusion

In her work on fairytales, Warner (1995, p. 411) argues that fairytales offer:

> a way of putting questions, of testing the structure as well as guaranteeing its safety, of thinking up alternatives as well as living daily reality in an examined way … For what is applauded and who sets the terms of the recognition and acceptance are always in question. Nor are the measure and weight of those terms assigned fixed values; unlike the statutory yards and metres kept safe in government vaults, they can and do change. Creating and contributing to the inhabited culture is not just a matter of individual creative genius, the

exceptional masterwork. We, the audience, you, the reader, are part of the story's future as well, its patterns are rising under the pressure of your palms, our fingers too.

The 'new fable', which draws on collaboratively constructed, arts-based knowledge, could take lessons from the marvellous, transformative and shifting ground that fairytales occupy. Assessing the validity of this knowledge is a collaborative affair and one that circumvents 'the entire, well-worn social science debates around "truth", validity and objectivity in which disembodied "snap shots" of individual's lives are commonly appropriated for dissection in the academic lab' (Inckle 2010, p. 38). Arts-based inquiry forms 'in the tension between *truthfulness* and *artistic integrity*' (Finley 2008; italics in the original) and to gauge its success involves coming up with ways of 'knowing the indistinct and the slippery without trying to grasp and hold them tight' (Law 2004, p. 3). Taking an alternative approach to assessing the worth of arts-based research impels us to reflect on what we are trying to achieve through our research and think creatively about how best to measure its impact: 'The question shifts from "Is this good arts-based research?" to "What is this arts-based research good for?"' (Leggo 2008, cited in Leavy 2009, p. 17).

Arts-based inquiry lends itself to contemplative thinking (Walsh et al. 2015), which means it can come close to acknowledging the 'profound sense of mystery' which remains even after 'the entire world has been transformed on the basis of scientific knowledge into a hierarchical structure of ever-widening systems' (Chaudhuri 1974, p. 195). Arts-based inquiry also has the ability to move us at an emotional and sensual level and have an impact on our thinking (Gunaratnam 2009, p. 26). Aesthetic evaluation thus needs to be based on the success of its pedagogical functions (Leavy 2009, p. 17). The work has to be accessible by those who share our goals and certainly 'must not be confined to intellectual elites' (Wolf 1993, p. 119). Given that people are 'as much persuaded by images, by mythology, and by poetry as they are by rational argumentation' (Johnson, cited in Kester 2004, p. 80), arts-based research has the advantage here. This requires a researcher who does not hide behind the illusion of objectivity, but rather believes that 'an emotionally vulnerable, linguistically evocative, and sensuously poetic voice can place us closer to the subjects we study' (Pelias 2004, p. 11, cited in Inckle 2010, p. 38). It also requires interrogating taken-for-granted assumptions, be they personal or cultural (Barone 2001). Most importantly, it requires the development of relationships and a sense of pleasure in the research process:

> The sharing of joy, whether physical, emotional, psychic, or intellectual, forms a bridge between the sharers which can be the basis for understanding much of what is not shared between them, and lessens the threat of their difference.
>
> (Lorde 2000, p. 4)

Chapter 8 develops this idea in its much more spirited take on the paradoxes and challenges of conducting arts-based, social justice-oriented research. These tensions can be seen as a game rather than a battle. The 'wisest thing ... [fairytale taught us] is to meet the forces of the mythical world with cunning and with high spirits' (Benjamin 1969/2006, p. 374).

8   The last laugh

Reality divided by reason always leaves a remainder.

(Haridas Chaudhuri 1974, p. 195)

The arts-based methodology described in this book involves moving away from a 'reasoned', rational approach to knowledge production. As Chaudhuri expresses, this is not sufficient in terms of capturing the less tangible elements of life. The artist Leonora Carrington declared that 'There are things that are not sayable. That is why we have art'. Employing the arts in collaborative research with marginalised groups offers much scope for producing knowledge that explores the unsaid, the mystery of day-to-day life, in ways that are engaging and moving. This book has documented a wide range of examples that do just this, including performed stories and digital stories, poetry and photovoice, metaphorical photographs, collage, dance and drama. It has been suggested that this research can be best understood through a theoretical framework that draws from critical theory, feminism and postmodernism. In order to promote social justice there is a need to recognise that knowledge is inseparable from issues of power and control (Foucault 1977). It is the 'knowers' that hold the power (Cohen-Mitchell 2000, p. 149) and some kinds of knowers are more acknowledged than others, just as some kinds of knowledge are held in higher esteem than others. The book has queried the claims that participatory and arts-based researchers frequently make regarding 'empowering' participants. Yet, whilst power cannot simply be 'handed over' through the research process, opportunities can be created for people to explore their own lives, to acknowledge their suffering, to communicate it and perhaps even to move forwards from it.

Polly Young-Eisendrath's (1997) work brings together psychoanalysis, with particular emphasis on Jung, and Buddhism as she writes about the 'gifts' that suffering and pain bring. Carl Jung, for instance, employed the alchemical metaphor of transforming lead into gold in this context. Buddhism meanwhile teaches that 'life is suffering' but the discomfort this causes can be alleviated through renouncing the need for control and addressing our self-protectiveness and the separateness we feel from others. Through this process exist possibilities for enriching transformations; for the creation of insight, compassion and renewal rather than a spiralling into more suffering. Of course, this in no way suggests that the poverty, oppression and stigma that so many marginalised people experience should be excused – but rather that there is, even within trauma, the possibility of finding some hope and meaning, of suffering leading to meanings that 'unlock the mystery of life' (ibid., p. 22).

Traditional forms of social inquiry truncate the possibilities for sharing stories, for engendering empathy and for encouraging transformative creativity. Collaborative, arts-based practice (whilst it should certainly not be billed as a social or psychological panacea) involves working closely together with others in inventive ways, and through this process provides a possibility of promoting self-compassion and compassion for others. This is knowledge that comes from witnessing suffering and it is here that 'deep and true creativity is born' (Young-Eisendrath 1997, p. 59). Of course, in research for social justice, the stories told do not always make for easy listening. There can, in stories of pain, be 'a gulf that cannot be overcome by empathy' (Ahmed 2004, p. 37) but that require a 'different kind of inhabitance'. Such stories operate as a political call to action: they are a call based on 'learning that we live with and beside each other, and yet we are not as one' (ibid., p. 39).

The imagination plays an important role in this process. It elicits 'human questioning, responses to blank spaces in experience, resistances to meaninglessness' (Greene 2000, p. 6). Yet as has been discussed, the imagination can also conjure up dark and diseased visions that do little to engender positive change. This is one of the many inconsistencies that the methods and projects discussed throughout the book have raised. Other tensions include the risk of research participants telling the stories that they think researchers and audiences want to hear; the very real possibility of perpetuating stereotypes; the discomfort that can arise when challenging stories are told; and audiences only hearing what they are able to deal with. These issues are important to acknowledge, not least because they communicate 'important messages about the complexity of everyday life' (O'Neill et al. 2002, p. 76). They are messy, contradictory, and at times politically questionable, but simultaneously rich and worthwhile, pulling hard at significant ideas about what knowledge is and what it means to be human.

The performative orientation of arts-based inquiry invites a richer and more nuanced exploration of humanity than much conventional research is able to provide. The openness that is required through this way of working means that rather than being forced 'to join dialogues the parameters of which are already fixed', researchers are invited into 'passionate inquiry' (Gergen and Gergen 2010, para. 11). This involves building respectful relationships and *enjoying* the work. There is pleasure to be had through this process (Foster 2012b). In order to communicate arts-based knowledge, language and imagery are put to full use and might include irony, metaphor, humour, and more (Gergen and Gergen 2010, para. 9). This chapter, rather than acting as a conventional conclusion, focuses on the joy and levity that are necessary to the research process itself and to the communication of findings. In so doing it provides a final 'statement' of the book's epistemological and methodological position. Echoes of mirth from earlier chapters resound: in Chapter 1, Radha's refusal to cook for her family leads to her throwing her head back and roaring with laughter; Chapter 3 opens with Carter's (1984) character, Fevvers, slapping her thigh and guffawing uproariously; in Chapter 6 my Sure Start colleagues, in carnivalesque fashion, rely on bawdy and irreverent humour.

There is defiance in this laughter and even a single gesture of defiance can pave the way for change and give impetus to any social movement (Singh 2009, p. 1). Weitz (2001, p. 670) agrees that individual acts of resistance offer the potential to spark social change and, in the long run, to shift the balance of power between social groups. One of the themes of this book has been the enmeshment of the personal with the political. In Radha's case, her refusal to cook that day challenges the profound gender inequality around the globe that means that domestic drudgery falls to women. The women at Sure Start challenge the ideology that underscores the entire initiative: that poor working-class mothers lack the ability to parent effectively (Foster 2015). The use of the arts to convey these messages touches audiences in ways that a more rationalist presentation cannot hope to. It is in arts-based presentation that research can 'become most alive' (Gunaratnam 2009, p. 14). This is not *just* about conveying knowledge or information:

> Art is not just an ornament or style used to make data more palatable or consumable. Art may well have meanings or messages but what makes it *art* is not content but its *affect*, the sensible force or style through which it produces content. Why, for example, would we spend two hours in the cinema watching a film if all we wanted were the story or the moral message?
> (Colebrook 2002, cited in Thompson 2009, p. 117)

The arts thus assist the aim that social inquiry should not only address injustice and suffering, but should also bring joy. The first section in this chapter, 'Wonder', advocates accordingly the need to remain open to the beauty and pleasure of life as we enjoy a curiosity about the world in which we live. It also suggests maintaining a sense of humour through this process. The next section, 'In jest', continues this line of argument. The rebellious, anarchic aspects of humour are the focus here. Examples of performance, dance and clowning enable discussion of the potential and the limits of such foolery. The final section, 'Celebration', meanwhile, looks at a research project that provides a playful take on 'forum theatre' with children in Brazil. It argues the need for frivolity in research, because 'if human inquiry is not exciting, life enhancing, even pleasurable, then what is it worth?' (Reason 2000, p. 6).

Wonder

Marina Warner (1995, p. xvi) describes how the verb 'to wonder' communicates both 'the receptive state of marvelling as well as the active desire to know, to inquire'. Whilst for Warner, this provides a useful definition of two substantive characteristics of the fairy tale – 'pleasure in the fantastic, curiosity about the real' (ibid.), it is similarly useful for describing the qualities of arts-based social research and the stories that are spun about people's lives. These stories, whether they are visual or performed, poetic or musical, provide the interested, attentive listener with a heightened appreciation of that everyday existence in which we are all enmeshed. This requires taking a different and perhaps unfamiliar perspective, eschewing conformity and understanding 'our givens as contingencies'. Doing so prevents habitual, predictable daily experiences or common sense being allowed to 'swathe everything' and swallow 'any hint of an opening possibility'. Instead there are choices to be made (Greene 2000, p. 23):

> [O]ne day the 'why' arises and everything begins in that weariness tinged with amazement. 'Begins' – this is important. Weariness comes at the end of the acts of a mechanical life, but at the same time it inaugurates the impulse of consciousness.
>
> (Camus 1955, p. 13, cited in Greene 2000, p. 24)

Alternative inquiry, research that refuses to 'toe the line of an orthodoxy which is in *many* ways quite illusory', enables this spark of possibility. It encourages people 'to be who they are', rather than to attempt to make themselves into something they are not 'but which is more easily observable, or countable, or manipulable' (Reason and Rowan 1981, pp. xxiii–xxiv). Working in a collaborative way that respects people's experiences and listens to their stories requires surrendering to uncertainty and remaining open to possibility. There are new avenues we might explore with the hope that they might lead to fresh terrain – although a sense of threat may lurk behind such a departure from established routes. Stray from the path, fairytales tell us, and 'shaggy branches tangle about you, trapping the unwary traveller in nets as if the vegetation itself were in a plot with the wolves who live there' (Carter 1996, p. 212). Face these fears though, in a defiant refusal to retread old ground, and new possibilities emerge. There is potential, not necessarily for living 'happily ever after', but for things to subtly change for the better, especially if we recognise the relationship between personal stories and wider society (Warner 1995, p. xvii). Developing a consciousness of the personal as political also stops us from personalising failure and enables a grasping of the complex interconnected dimensions of oppression (Ledwith and Springett 2010, p. 28).

Marginalised groups are consistently represented, and more often than not misrepresented, by others. The arts offer a way of working with such communities and respecting their ways of living. Involving people in the research process has the potential to enable them to determine their own social and political realities, and can restore a social bond through a collective understanding of meaning. In Freirean terms, this is a praxis that involves collective and *creative* participation. It is creative in the sense that that our 'human situation' means we are not only able to see the world as it is, but also as it could be (Crotty 1998, p. 149). There is a possibility here for joy to play a part in this process of envisioning a better world. Russian-American anarchist Emma Goldman discusses her radicalism:

I did not believe that a Cause which stood for a beautiful ideal, for anarchism, for release and freedom from conventions and prejudice, should demand the denial of life and joy. I insisted that our Cause could not expect me to become a nun and that the movement would not be turned into a cloister. If it meant that, I did not want it. 'I want freedom, expression, everybody's right to beautiful, radiant things.' Anarchism meant that to me, and I would live it in spite of the whole world ...

(Goldman 2006, p. 42, cited in Thompson 2009, p. 1)

James Thomson (2009, p. 2), in a book that celebrates the resistant qualities of performance whilst at the same time acknowledging its capacity for pleasure, introduces two ideas that he takes from Goldman's work: first, that art enables people to tolerate suffering, not so that they become immune to it, but so that they have the energy to continue to resist; second, that participation in the joyful is not a diversion from reality, but rather part of a dream of a 'beautiful' future, in the sense that it becomes an inspirational force.

The world itself, regarded through a performative lens on reality, might be seen as an active entity, displacing the passive 'logic of "discovery"' with 'a power-charged social relation of "conversation"' (Haraway 1991, p. 198). If the agency of the world is acknowledged, it might introduce 'unsettling possibilities', including 'a sense of the world's independent sense of humour' (ibid., p. 199). Rather than being a resource for human kind, the world could be seen as 'witty agent' or a 'coding trickster with whom we must learn to converse' (ibid.). There is a need then to look at the 'feminist discards from the Western deck of cards, to look for the trickster figures that might turn a stacked deck into a potent set of wild cards, jokers, for refiguring possible worlds' (ibid., p. 4).

In jest

Anna Deavere Smith's performance piece, *Fires in the Mirror*, is based on the Crown Heights riots in Brooklyn, a series of violent tensions between the Black and Jewish communities which were sparked by the accidental killing of a young Black boy by a car driven by a Jewish man. Smith carried out a number of interviews after the event with major players including leading politicians, religious leaders and local residents. She worked the transcripts verbatim into a series of monologues which she performed herself, taking on the roles of the characters interviewed. Smith's portrayal of these figures is unsettling, mediated as they are through her Black female identity. In West's (1993, p. xviii) foreword to the published version of Smith's work, he remarks on the humour involved:

Her funny characterizations – that for some border on caricatures – provoke genuine laughter even as we know that laughter is an inadequate response to the pain, cruelty and sheer absurdity of the crisis.

The performance can be understood as both 'illuminating and limiting'. The various speeches 'create competing and contradictory narratives that make it difficult for the audience to take sides or to form a united community sure of where justice lies' (Jay 2007, p. 120). It is this sense of uncertainty that typifies arts-based and aesthetic ways of knowing. Claiming this as 'research' is 'an act of rebellion against the monolithic "truth" that science is supposed to entail' (Finley 2008, p. 73). There is an acknowledgement that there is more than one story to be told, especially by 'invisible' individuals or groups, rather than one monolithic common national history (Osler and Zhu 2011, p. 231). The arts are on the margin, that 'place for those feelings and intuitions which daily life doesn't have a place for and mostly seems to suppress ... With the arts, people can make a space for themselves and fill it with intimations of freedom and presence' (Donoghue, cited in Greene 2000, p. 28). Humour throws another layer of rebellion, of uncertainty and unease into the mix. It might act as a form of resistance to power and inequality through its reliance on 'a kind of "double vision" – the ability to see the absurdity, irony or double meanings in social situations and roles' (MacLure 2009, p. 108).

Warner (2000) describes Josephine Baker's banana costume for her notorious performance in the *Revue Nègre* of 1926 to a predominantly White audience. Topless, save for several strings of pearls, she wears a belt fashioned from hanging bananas, 'a scanty parody of a Hawaiian hula skirt' (ibid., p. 364). The dance involved her entering a staged jungle, crawling along a fallen tree trunk on all fours and then launching into a vigorous dance on behalf of a sleeping young White man that she comes across. The bananas bounced as she embodied the 'spirit of the jungle', the 'untamed, unfettered libido' (ibid.). Yet she also 'spoofed the expectation of it' and laughed joyously at the folly of the audience in her inhabitation of 'the fool's double consciousness, the ironic cynicism that turns all appearances unstable' (ibid., p. 366). In the end, Warner surmises, Baker remains a spectacle that is unable to resist commodification and alienation: 'her wit, her energy, her mischief, her resplendent self-fabrication meet that stone wall of mass media culture, its feeding on stereotype, and her joy freezes in the gaze of racial ascriptions' (ibid.). Once again, the paradox of the carnivalesque can be seen at play. The possibility of change, the inversion of power relations, is often fleeting and transient.

The carnival 'challenges the pompous and the authoritative; it reduces the grandiose to size; it makes holes in empty pieties' (Greene 2000, p. 63). Yet, as one of Angela Carter's subversive characters points out, there are 'limits to the power of laughter' (Webb 1994, p. 306). The carnival is not able to 'rewrite history, undo the effects of war or alter what is happening on the news'. However, it does offer a 'tantalising promise' of how things might be 'if we altered the conditions that tie us down' (ibid.). This is why the 'creative things that make it up in life are so precious: laughter, sex and art' (ibid., p. 307). Involvement in creative and fun-filled activities spills over into other areas of life. Seeley, for instance, describes beautifully how everyday life is enriched by her engagement with the art form of clowning (Seeley and Reason 2008, p. 44). She notes how the lingering effects of her clowning practice infiltrate the day-to-day:

Simple encounters like buying fuel on the way home, or chatting at the supermarket checkout temporarily take on new significance and delight. People entering through doors seem to be 'making an entrance' or 'doing a crossing' and I notice greater richness in the everyday gestures and eye contact which otherwise I might miss ... It's as if the heightened awareness of the clown energy calls forth greater engagement and playfulness in others. For me this evokes a feeling of shared humanity, a playful twinkle in the eye, a meta-communication about this being human which I associate strongly with our species-level need to find compassionate ways of living that are less destructive, less acquisitive, more just and more in tune with the worlds of which we are a part.

Fremeaux and Ramsden (2007, p. 25) draw parallels between the practice of rebel clowning, a form of radical activism that draws on the ancient art of clowning, and carnival: both are 'rooted in a blurring of the distinction between art and life'. The Clandestine Insurgent Rebel Clown Army in the UK takes part in political demonstrations but in ways which have ended in hugs with the police rather than violence, the clowns having drawn smiley faces with lipstick on police shields. On other occasions, clowns have been searched by the police resulting in some of them collapsing in hysterical giggles because they are ticklish and others having so many layers of clothing that it takes an age to strip them down to their stripy underwear. Given that police and army strategy is based on predictability and understanding the 'enemy's next move', this is unsettling. Rebel clowning thus provides an 'exploration of authoritarianism through parody and ridicule' (ibid., p. 23). This is in line with the long history of the clown or fool as trickster, healer or shaman figures who have long held the critical social function of healing and critiquing through disruption. The arts have a way of radiating through our 'variously lived worlds' and, in so doing, expose not only the darks and the lights, but also the 'wounds and the scars and the healed places, the empty containers and the overflowing ones, the faces ordinarily lost in the crowds' (Greene 2000, p. 29).

Celebration

Research for social justice can be a celebratory affair. It does not need to be dry and dour. There is so much to learn from exploring the world, even the profound injustices that exist, through collective and joyful processes. Nogueira et al.'s (2014) work provides an example of playfulness in social inquiry. This involved a performance project with children in a community in Forianópolis that aimed to combine the strengths of 'forum theatre', and its emphasis on challenging oppression, with the Brazilian popular tradition of the *Boi de Mamão*. This is a lighthearted celebration of music, dance and acting that centres around the death and resurrection of the bull (Video 20). Given that forum theatre can be construed as rigid in regard to its adherence to a set of rules, the practitioners hoped that incorporating themes from the *Boi de Mamão* would breathe new life into it. Thus they created *The Forum of the Bull*.

The main characters of the *Boi de Mamão* are Mateus (Matthew), the owner of the bull, and Vaqueiro (Cowboy), who takes care of the bull. They are supported by a host of quirky and fantastical characters, including a bernúncia, a sort of Chinese dragon, and Maricota, a huge doll with very long arms. The caller tells the story, in the most part through song, and directs each character to the centre of the circle in which the action happens. Mateus and Vaqueiro are always in the circle and act out the caller's words. They are 'cheerful clowns, pranksters and communicators' (Nogueira et al. 2014, p. 185) and thus the practitioners draw on the tradition of 'fooling' in the theatre and evoke the figure of the joker from Boal's forum theatre (see Chapter 5). *The Forum of the Bull* required a joker that had an in-depth knowledge of the *Boi de Mamão* and of the local community, as well as an ability to listen to spectators' contributions, connecting 'representation and reality' without suppressing the playfulness of the *Boi de Mamão* tradition. At the same time there was a need to remain true to the original role of the fool or trickster, in terms of exposing the contradictions and ironies underpinning the status quo.

A series of games was carried out with the participants by the joker. One involved an examination of the oppression that exists between employer and employee (in this case between Mateus and Vaqueiro). One group of participants acted as Mateus, the other as Vaqueiro. After beginning with an opening song, the participants were required to think about the possibility of Vaqueiro being employed in the task of caring for the cattle. Mateus poses the question: how much do you want to get? The participants spent time working on the answer to this question. Initially they answered that they would like food and a place to sleep, but the joker pointed out that this amounted to slave labour. Together they developed the idea of a salary and the necessities for living a full life including housing, health and education. A song was written that incorporated these proposals:

I want a little bit to buy my house,
I want another bit to have good health,
Give me a little more to get fed.
Pay with my wage to get a good school.
Oh *Mateus*, oh *Mateus*,
Do not be so greedy
I'll take care of your bull, oh Matthew
And I deserve a few coins.
Mateus' song:
With the amount I give, you can buy a tile;
With the amount I give, you can buy an aspirin;
With the wages I give, you can buy lunch.
The minimum wage will even buy a notebook;
Oh *Vaqueiro*, oh *Vaqueiro*,
Listen well to what I tell you,
You will take care of my bull, oh Vaqueiro
And I'll give you a decent income.

In the context of applied theatre (but this might apply to any arts-based work), Prentki (2009b, p. 367) argues that the most effective practice is one that combines the post-Enlightenment notion of social improvement with the medieval one of community carnival. This results in 'a folly of social intervention' (ibid.) orchestrated by a practitioner who is at the same time both social worker and fool, and who, through highlighting absurdity and contradiction, offers alternative possibilities. There is an importance in valuing these accomplishments, because: 'In the sharing of successes, however small and micro, we gain courage and encouragement to learn by doing' (Maguire 1996, p. 38); this requires 'joyful affirmation' of our strengths and perhaps even enables us to redefine success (ibid.). Such shared pleasure builds valuable connections between people. This process is paradoxical in that as we unite, we develop a greater appreciation of what is *different* about each other, and about our experiences of this life.

Conclusion

There are multiple approaches to knowledge production, and acknowledging this raises a challenge to the dominant master narrative: 'Any practice which claims to be predicated on equality and social justice has to heed these diverse ways of knowing and being in the world' (Ledwith and Springett 2010, p. 109). Listening to a variety of stories from a variety of people provides opportunities to acknowledge and potentially rectify wide-ranging cases of discrimination and oppression (Osler and Zhu 2011, p. 231). Even having shared experiences in common does not necessarily mean that they will be 'felt' in the same way:

> So we may walk into the room and 'feel the atmosphere,' but what we may feel depends on the angle of our arrival. Or we may say that the atmosphere is already angled; it is always felt from a specific point.
>
> (Ahmed 2010, p. 37)

For Eisner (2008b, p. 22), arts-based research 'is the result of artistically crafting the description of the situation so that it can be seen from another angle'. Traditional research has advocated the practice of triangulation in order to understand issues from more than one perspective. Richardson (1998, p. 358), however, proposes that in postmodernist mixed-genre texts, the metaphor of the crystal is much more pertinent than that of the triangle, since it is recognised that there are myriad ways of viewing the world (and we should not be limited to just three angles). Crystals are 'prisms that reflect externalities and refract within themselves, creating different colours, patterns, arrays, casting off in different directions. What we see depends on our angle of repose' (ibid.). This metaphor has much resonance for the work described in this book. It takes into account a variety of standpoints, as well as capturing the complexities, the beauty and the 'magic' of life. The research process itself can be understood as a work of art, an aesthetic experience (Janesick 1998).

Ultimately, 'the story told is the dance in all its complexity, context, originality, and passion' (Janesick 1998, p. 53). Les Back (2007, p. 3) employs the metaphor of dance in relation to sociology:

> I started to view sociology as part of an embrace with and connection to the dance of life with all its heavy and cumbersome steps. It is an aspiration to hold the experience of others in your arms while recognizing that what we touch is always moving, unpredictable, irreducible and mysteriously opaque.

Embracing the dance of life, demonstrating a 'willingness to live in the realm of mythology, metaphor, and mystery' (Rankin 2015, p. 78) is a radical move. It means eschewing the certainty and knowledge that science claims to provide. Science has helped us to understand more about how the world works, but a less welcome aspect of this technical information is that we have lost the acceptance of ambiguity and doubt. Moreover, scientific understandings of the world tend to be compartmentalised. Whilst in some indigenous cultures it is understood that everything is connected, from people to animals, plants, water, the oceans and the mountains, in the Western world we have 'come to believe that we are connected to nothing' (ibid.). Losing this insight poses much risk for human kind as well as for the planet.

Arts-based researchers must focus on the promise that artful representations have the capacity to provoke both reflective dialogue and meaningful action and, thereby, to change the world in positive ways that contribute to progressive, participatory, and ethical social action (Finley 2008, p. 75). Knowledge, even radical knowledge, requires 'sensibility and sensuality' in its production, otherwise all we are left with is a 'cold, unfeeling shell of breathing flesh devoid of the capacity for love, suffering, joy and compassion' (Shapiro 1999, p. 161). A hands-on, creative and participative approach to social inquiry avoids producing alienated knowledge, apparently devoid of any socio-political or interpersonal context. In order to move towards transformative action that celebrates freedom and dignity, the quest for social justice needs to be combined with such qualities as love, compassion and humility. These must be understood 'not as feelings or even ideas but as actual practices' (Fernandes 2003, p. 59).

The book has argued that if we are to know the world differently then we need to 'act and be differently' (Maguire 1996, p. 31) in the world. We need to 'be kind' (see Chapter 7) and compassionate in our everyday behaviours and interactions with others so that we are not reproducing the inequalities and exclusions that we speak out against. This is one of the most significant values of employing the arts in research. They have the ability to open us up to one another in ways that highlight our vulnerabilities. When we lose our tolerance for vulnerability, joy becomes foreboding (Brown 2012). In other words, fear of exposing ourselves to loss or failure can prevent us truly living and interacting with the wonders of the world. Richard Quinney's (1998, p. xv) 'ethnography of everyday life', a document of ten years of the writer's life, ends with 'a requiem for the living and the dead'. This requiem acts as a meditation on life: what has gone before and what remains: 'Even as we live this moment, a requiem is playing in the background. A music that assures us that we live, and a music that makes us grateful for this life. This everyday and wondrous life' (ibid.). There are no certainties in this world; life twists and turns, and research practice needs to pay heed to such individually experienced, relationally mediated, socially embedded complexity. Indeed, a truly transformative research practice requires a careful listening for the music that accompanies our dance through life, the harmonies and beats that sing and pulsate through our suffering and joy.

References

Abbott, Pamela and Wallace, Claire (1998) Health visiting, social work, nursing and midwifery: A history. In Pamela Abbott and Liz Meerabeau (eds) *The Sociology of the Caring Professions*, 2nd edn, pp. 20–53. London: UCL Press.

Ahmed, Sara (2004) *The Cultural Politics of Emotion.* Edinburgh: Edinburgh University Press.

Ahmed, Sara (2010) *The Promise of Happiness.* Durham, NC and London: Duke University Press.

Albergato-Muterspaw, Francesca and Fenwick, Tara (2007) Passion and politics through song: Recalling music to the arts-based debates in adult education. In Clover, Darlene E. and Stalker, Joyce (eds) *The Arts and Social Justice: Re-crafting Adult Education and Community Cultural Leadership* pp. 147–164. Leicester: NIACE.

Allen, Quaylan (2012) Photographs and stories: Ethics, benefits and dilemmas of using participant photography with Black middle-class male youth. *Qualitative Research* 12 (4): 443–458.

Allman, Paula (2001) *Critical Education Against Global Capitalism: Karl Marx and Revolutionary Education.* Westport, CT: Bergin and Harvey.

Almack, Kathryn (2003) Interview: Beverley Skeggs. *BSA Network*, 86, pp. 2–5.

Anzaldúa, Gloria (1987) *Borderlands/La Frontera: The New Mestiza.* San Fransisco: Aunt Lute Books.

Archibald, Jo-Ann (2008) *Indigenous Storywork: Educating the Heart, Mind, Body and Spirit.* Vancouver: University of British Columbia Press.

Arts Council England (2014) *The Value of Arts and Culture to People and Society: An Evidence Review.* Manchester: Arts Council England.

Austin, Deborah A. (1996) Kaleidoscope: The same and different. In Ellis, Carolyn and Bochner, Arthur P. (eds) *Composing Ethnography: Alternative Forms of Qualitative Writing* pp. 206–230. Walnut Creek, CA: AltaMira Press.

Austin, Diane and Forinash, Michele (2005). Arts-based research. In Wheeler, Barbara L. (ed.), *Music Therapy Research*, 2nd edn, pp. 458–471. Gilsum, NH: Barcelona.

Auther, Elissa (2009) *String, Felt, Thread: The Hierarchy of Art and Craft in American Art.* Minneapolis: University of Minnesota Press

Back, Les (2007) *The Art of Listening.* Oxford: Berg.

Bagley, Carl and Cancienne, Mary Beth (2002) Educational research and intertextual forms of (re)presentation: The case for dancing the data. In Bagley, Carl and Cancienne, Mary Beth (eds) *Dancing the Data* pp. 3–19. New York: Peter Lang.

Bagley, Carl (2008) Educational ethnography as performance art: Towards a sensuous feeling and knowing. *Qualitative Research* 8 (1): 53–72.

Bakhtin, Mikhail (1968/1984) *Rabelais and His World* (translated by Hélène Iswolsky). Bloomington, IN: Indiana University Press.

Bakhtin, Mikhail (1984) *Problems of Dostoevsky's Poetics* (translated by Caryl Emerson). Minneapolis: University of Minnesota Press.

Ballengee-Morris, Christine (2008) Indigenous aesthetics: Universal Circles related and connected to everything called life. *Art Education* 61 (2): 30–33.

Banks, Sarah and Rifkin, Frances with Davidson, Heather, Holmes, Claire and Moore, Niamh (2014) Performing ethics: Using participatory theatre to explore ethical issues in community-based participatory research. Durham: Centre for Social Justice and Community Action, Durham University.

Barone, Tom (2001) Science, art, and the predispositions of educational researchers. *Educational Researcher* 30 (7): 24–28.

Barone, Tom (2008) How arts-based research can change minds. In Cahnmann-Taylor, Melisa and Siegesmund, Richard (eds) *Arts-Based Research in Education* pp. 28–49. New York: Routledge.

Barone, Tom and Eisner, Elliott W. (2012) *Arts Based Research*. London: Sage.

Basting, Anne Davis (2001) 'God is a talking horse': Dementia and the performance of self. *The Drama Review* 45 (3): 78–94.

Basu, Purabi (1999) French leave. In Ganguly, Swati and Dutta Gupta, Sarmistha (translators and eds) *The Stream Within: Short Stories by Contemporary Bengali Women* pp. 9–14. Calcutta: Bhatkal Books.

Becker, Howard (2007) *Telling About Society*. Chicago: University of Chicago Press.

Behar, Ruth (2003) Ethnography and the book that was lost. *Ethnography* 4(1): 15–39.

Behar, Ruth (2008) Between poetry and anthropology. In Cahnmann-Taylor, Melisa and Siegesmund, Richard (eds) *Arts-Based Research in Education* pp. 55–71. New York: Routledge.

Benjamin, Walter (1969/2006) The storyteller: Reflections on the works of Nikolai Leskov. In Hale, Dorothy J. (ed.) *The Novel: An Anthology of Criticism and Theory 1900–2000* pp. 361–378. Malden, MA: Blackwell.

Beresford, Peter (2002) User involvement in research and evaluation: Liberation or regulation? *Social Policy and Society* 1 (2): 95–105.

Berger, John (1972) *Ways of Seeing*. London: BBC Books/Pelican.

Bhattacharya, Kakali (2008) Voices lost and found: Using found poetry in qualitative research. In Cahnmann-Taylor, Melisa and Siegesmund, Richard (eds) *Arts-Based Research in Education* pp. 83–88. New York: Routledge.

Bhattacharyya, Gargi (1998) *Tales of Dark-skinned Women: Race, Gender and Global Culture*. London: UCL Press.

Bishop, Claire (2006) The social turn: Collaboration and its discontents. *Artforum* February: 178–183.

Bishop, Claire (2012) *Artificial Hells: Participatory Art and the Politics of Spectatorship*. London: Verso.

Boal, Augusto (1979) *Theater of the Oppressed*. New York: Theatre Communications Group.

Bochner, Arthur P. (2000) Criteria against ourselves. *Qualitative Inquiry* 6 (2): 266–272.

Boler, Megan (1997) The risks of empathy: Interrogating multiculturalism's gaze. *Cultural Studies* 11 (2): 253–273.

Bourdieu, Pierre and Wacquant, Loïc (2001) NewLiberalSpeak: Notes on the new planetary vulgate. *Radical Philosophy* 105 (January/February): 2–5.

Bradbury, Hilary and Reason, Peter (2001) Conclusion: Broadening the bandwidth of validity: Issues and choice-points for improving the quality of action research. In Reason, Peter and Bradbury, Hilary (eds) *Handbook of Action Research* pp. 447–455. London: Sage.

Brecht, Bertolt (1977) *The Measures Taken and Other Lehrstücke*. London: Eyre Methuen.

Bresler, Liora (2008) The music lesson. In Knowles, J. Gary and Cole, Ardra L. (eds) *Handbook of the Arts in Qualitative Research: Perspectives, Methodologies, Examples, and Issues* pp. 226–237. Thousand Oaks, CA: Sage.

Broadwood, Jo with Bunting, Catherine, Andrews, Tom, Abrams, Dominic and Van de Vyver, Julie (2012) Arts and Kindness. Canterbury: People United Publishing.

Brooker, Peter (2003) *A Glossary of Cultural Theory*, 2nd edn. London: Arnold.

Brown, Brené (2012) *Daring Greatly*. London: Penguin.

Burns, Diane and Chantler, Khatidja (2011) Feminist methodologies. In Somekh, Bridget and Lewin, Cathy (eds) *Theory and Methods in Social Research* pp. 70–77. London: Sage.

Byrne, Anne and Lentin, Ronit (2000) Introduction: Feminist research methodologies in the social sciences. In Byrne, Anne and Lentin, Ronit (eds) *(Re)searching Women: Feminist Research Methodologies in the Social Sciences in Ireland* pp. 1–59. Dublin: Institute of Public Administration.

Cahnmann-Taylor, Melisa (2008) Arts-based research: Histories and new directions. In Cahnmann-Taylor, Melisa and Siegesmund, Richard (eds) *Arts-Based Research in Education* pp. 3–15. New York: Routledge.

Calvino, Italo (1997) *Invisible Cities*. London: Vintage.

Cancienne, Mary Beth and Bagley, Carl (2008) Dance as method: The process and product of movement. In Liamputtong, Pranee and Rumbold, Jean (eds) *Knowing Differently: Arts-Based and Collaborative Research Methods* pp. 169–187. New York: Nova.

Cancienne, Mary Beth and Snowber, Celeste N. (2003) Writing rhythm: Movement as method. *Qualitative Inquiry* 9 (2): 237–253.

Canepa, Nancy (2008) in Haase, Donald (ed.) *The Greenwood Encyclopedia of Folktales and Fairytales*, vol. 1 pp. 155–157. Westport, CT: Greenwood Press.

Capous-Desyllas, Moshoula (2015) Collage as reflexivity: Illustrations and reflections of a photovoice study with sex workers. In Wahab, Stéphanie, Anderson-Nathe, Ben and Gringeri, Christina (eds) *Feminisms in Social Work Research* pp. 189–208. Abingdon: Routledge.

Carey, Malcolm (2011). Should I stay or should I go? Practical, ethical and political challenges to 'service user' participation within social work research. *Qualitative Social Work* 10 (2): 224–243.

Carey, Malcolm (2013) More than this? Some ethical doubts (and possibilities) regarding service user and carer participation within spcial work. In Carey, Malcolm and Green, Lorraine (eds) *Practical Social Work Ehics: Complex Dilemmas Within Applied Social Care* pp. 199–226. Farnham, Surrey: Ashgate.

Carey, Malcolm and Foster, Victoria (2013) Social work, ideology, discourse and the limits of post-hegemony. *Journal of Social Work* 13 (3): 248–266.

Carr, Sarah (2004). Has service user participation made a difference to social care services? *SCIE Position Paper 3*. London: SCIE/Policy Press.

Carr, Sarah (2007). Participation, power, conflict and change: Theorizing dynamics of service user participation in the social care system of England and Wales. *Critical Social Policy* 27(2): 266–276.

Carter, Angela (1985) *Nights at the Circus*. London: Picador.

Carter, Angela (1993) *Expletives Deleted: Selected Writings*. London: Vintage.

Carter, Angela (1994) In Pantoland. In Carter, Angela, *American Ghosts and Old World Wonders* pp. 98–109. London: Vintage.

Carter, Angela (1996) The company of wolves. In Carter, Angela, *Burning Your Boats: Collected Short Stories* pp. 212–220. London: Vintage.

Castell, Sarah and Thompson, Julian (2007) Understanding attitudes to poverty in the UK: Getting the public's attention. York: Joseph Rowntree Foundation. www.jrf.org.uk/system/files/2000-poverty-attitudes-uk.pdf.

Chamberlayne, Prue and Smith, Martin (eds) (2009) *Art, Creativity and Imagination in Social Work Practice*. Abingdon: Routledge.

Chaplin, Elizabeth (1994) *Sociology and Visual Representation*. Abingdon: Routledge.

Chaplin, Elizabeth (2004) My visual diary. In Knowles, Caroline and Sweetman, Paul (eds) *Picturing the Social Landscape: Visual Methods and the Sociological Imagination* pp. 35–48. London: Routledge.

Chaplin, Elizabeth (2005) The photograph in theory. *Sociological Research Online* 10 (1): www.socresonline.org.uk/10/1/chaplin.html

Chaudhuri, Haridas (1974) *Being, Evolution, and Immortality*. Wheaton, IL: Theosophical Publishing House.

Chekhov, Anton (1999) The kiss. In Ford, Richard (ed.) *The Essential Tales of Chekhov*. London: Granta.

Clapp, Susannah (2012) *Postcards from Angela Carter*. London: Bloomsbury.

Clark, Andrew (2013) Haunted by images? Ethical moments and anxieties in visual research. *Methodological Innovations Online* 8 (2): 68–81.

Clark, Katerina and Holquist, Michael (1984) *Mikhail Bakhtin*. Cambridge, MA: Harvard University Press.

Clarke, Karen (2006) Childhood, parenting and early intervention: A critical examination of the Sure Start national programme. *Critical Social Policy* 26 (4): 699–721.

Clifford, James (1986) On ethnographic allegory. In Clifford, James and Marcus, George E. (eds) *Writing Culture: The Poetics and Politics of Ethnography* pp. 98–121. Berkeley, CA: University of California Press.

Clifford, James (1988) *The Predicament of Culture: Twentieth Century Ethnography, Literature and Art*. Cambridge, MA: Harvard University Press.

Clover, Darlene E. (2005) Sewing stories and acting activism: Women's leadership and learning through drama and craft. *Ephemera* 5 (4): 629–642.

Clover, Darlene E. (2007) Tapestries through the making. In Clover, Darlene E. and Stalker, Joyce (eds) *The Arts and Social Justice: Re-crafting Adult Education and Community Cultural Leadership* pp. 83–101. Leicester: NIACE.

Clover, Darlene E. (2011) Successes and challenges of feminist arts-based participatory methodologies with homeless/street-involved women in Victoria. *Action Research* 9 (1): 12–26.

Clover, Darlene E. and Stalker, Joyce (2007) Introduction. In Clover, Darlene E. and Stalker, Joyce (eds) *The Arts and Social Justice: Re-crafting Adult Education and Community Cultural Leadership* pp. 1–18. Leicester: NIACE.

Cohen-Mitchell, Joanie B. (2000). Disabled women in El Salvador reframing themselves. In Truman, Carole, Mertens, Donna M. and Humphries, Beth (eds) *Research and Inequality* pp. 143–176. London: UCL Press.

Collins, Patricia Hill (1990) *Black Feminist Thought: Knowledge, Consciousness and the Politics of Empowerment*. Boston: Unwin Hyman.

Conquergood, Dwight (1991). Rethinking ethnography: Towards a critical cultural politics. *Communication Monographs* 58: 170–194.

Conquergood, Dwight (1993) Storied worlds and the work of teaching. *Communication Education* 42 (October): 337–348.

Conquergood, Dwight (2002) Performance studies: Interventions and radical research. *The Drama Review* 46 (2): 145–156.

Cook, Tina (2012) Where participatory approaches meet pragmatism in funded (health) research: The challenge of finding meaningful spaces. *Forum Qualitative Sozialforschung/Forum: Qualitative Social Research* 13 (1), Art. 18, http://nbn-resolving.de/urn:nbn:de:0114-fqs1201187.

Cowling, Jamie (ed.) (2004) *For Art's Sake*. London: IPPR.

Craig, Gary (2002) Poverty, social work and social justice. *British Journal of Social Work* 32 (6): 669–682.

Cribb, Alan and Gewirtz, Sharon (2003) Towards a sociology of just practices: An analysis of plural conceptions of justice. In Vincent, Carol (ed.) *Social Justice, Education and Identity* pp. 15–29. London: RoutledgeFalmer.

Crotty, Michael (1998) *The Foundations of Social Research*. London: Sage.

Danow, David K. (2004) *The Spirit of Carnival: Magical Realism and the Grotesque*. Lexington: The University Press of Kentucky.

Darts, David (2004) Visual culture jam: Art, pedagogy, and creative resistance. *Studies in Art Education* 45 (4): 313–327.

De Benedictis, Sara (2012) 'Feral' parents: Austerity parenting under neoliberalism *Studies in the Maternal* 4 (2): 1–21, www.mamsie.bbk.ac.uk.

Defilippis, Joseph Nicholas (2015) A letter to activists entering academia. In Wahab, Stephanie, Anderson-Nathe, Ben and Gringeri, Christina (eds) *Feminisms in Social Work Research* pp. 36–51. Abingdon: Routledge.

Denzin, Norman K. (1997) *Interpretive Ethnography: Ethnographic Practices for the 21st Century*. Thousand Oaks, CA: Sage.

Denzin, Norman K. (2000) Aesthetics and the practices of qualitative enquiry. *Qualitative Inquiry* 6: 256–265.

Denzin, Norman K. (2003) *Performance Ethnography: Critical Pedagogy and the Politics of Culture*. Thousand Oaks, CA: Sage.

Denzin, Norman K. and Giardina, Michael D. (2009) Introduction: Qualitative inquiry and social justice: Towards a politics of hope. In Denzin, Norman K. and Giardina, Michael D. (eds) *Qualitative Inquiry and Social Justice: Towards a Politics of Hope* pp. 11–50. Walnut Creek, CA: Left Coast Press.

Denzin, Norman K. and Giardina, Michael D. (2010) Introduction: The elephant in the living room, OR advancing the conversation about the politics of evidence. In Denzin, Norman K. and Giardina, Michael D. (eds) *Qualitative Inquiry and the Politics of Evidence* pp. 9–51. Walnut Creek, CA: Left Coast Press.

Denzin, Norman K. and Lincoln, Yvonna S. (2002) *The Qualitative Inquiry Reader*. Thousand Oaks, CA: Sage.

Denzin, Norman K. and Lincoln, Yvonna S. (2011) *The Sage Handbook of Qualitative Research*, 4th edn. Thousand Oaks, CA: Sage.

DeVault, Marjorie (1999) Talking back to Sociology. In De Vault, Marjorie, *Liberating Method*. Philadelphia, PA: Temple University Press.

Dezeen magazine (2012) Pont de Singe bridge by Olivier Grossetete. 15th November. http://www.dezeen.com/2012/11/15/pont-de-singe-balloon-bridge-by-olivier-grossetete/

Dockery, Grindl (2000) Participatory research: Whose roles, whose responsibilities? In Truman, Carole, Mertens, Donna M. and Humphries, Beth (eds) *Research and Inequality* pp. 95–110. London: UCL Press.

Dolan, Jill (2005) *Utopia in Performance: Finding Hope at the Theater.* Ann Arbor: University of Michigan Press.

Doucet, Andrea and Mauthner, Natasha S. (2006) Feminist methodologies and epistemologies. In Bryant, Clifton D. and Dennis L. Peck (eds) *Handbook of 21st Century Sociology* pp. 36–42. Thousand Oaks, CA: Sage.

Driessnack, Martha (2006) Draw-and-tell conversations with children about fear. *Qualitative Health Research* 16 (10): 1414–1435.

Dudley, Mary Jo (2003) The transformative power of video: Ideas, images, processes and outcomes. In White, Shirley A. (ed.) *Participatory Video: Images that Transform and Empower* pp. 145–156. New Delhi: Sage.

Eagleton, Terry (2000) *The Idea of Culture.* Oxford: Blackwell.

Eagleton, Terry (2004) *After Theory.* London: Penguin.

Eagleton, Terry (2007a) *Ideology: An Introduction.* London: Verso.

Eagleton, Terry (2007b) *How to Read a Poem.* Oxford: Blackwell.

Eisenhauer, Jennifer (2012) Behind closed doors: The pedagogy and interventionist practice of digital storytelling. *Journal of Curriculum and Pedagogy* 9: 7–15.

Eisner, Elliot W. (2001) Concerns and aspirations for qualitative research in the new millennium. *Qualitative Research* 1 (2): 135–145.

Eisner, Elliot W. (2008a) Art and knowledge. In Knowles, J. Gary and Cole, Ardra L. (eds) *Handbook of the Arts in Qualitative Research: Perspectives, Methodologies, Examples, and Issues* pp. 3–12. Thousand Oaks, CA: Sage.

Eisner, Elliot W. (2008b) Persistent tensions in arts-based research. In Cahnmann-Taylor, Melisa and Siegesmund, Richard (eds) *Arts-Based Research in Education* pp. 16–27. New York: Routledge.

Emmison, Michael, Smith, Philip D. and Mayall, Margery (2012) *Researching the Visual,* 2nd edn. London: Sage.

Etmanski, Catherine (2007) Voyeurism, consciousness-raising, empowerment: Opportunities and challenges of using legislative theatre to 'practise democracy'. In Clover, Darlene E. and Stalker, Joyce (eds) *The Arts and Social Justice: Re-crafting Adult Education and Community Cultural Leadership* pp. 105–124. Leicester: NIACE.

European Commission (2008) Scientific Evidence for Policy-Making. Brussels: European Commission Office.

Fawcett, Barbara, Featherstone, Brid and Goddard, Jim (2004) *Contemporary Child Care Policy and Practice.* Basingstoke: Palgrave Macmillan.

Fels, Lynn (2015) Woman overboard: Pedagogical moments of performative inquiry. In Walsh, Susan, Bickel, Barbara and Leggo, Carl (eds) *Arts-based and Contemplative Practices in Research and Teaching* pp. 112–123. New York and Abingdon: Routledge.

Fernandes, Leela (2003) *Transforming Feminist Practice: Non-Violence, Social Justice and the Possibilities of a Spiritualized Feminism.* San Fransisco: Aunt Lute Books.

Finley, Susan (2000) 'Dream Child': The role of poetic dialogue in homeless research. *Qualitative Inquiry* 6 (3): 432–434.

Finley, Susan (2008) Arts-based research. In Knowles, J. Gary and Cole, Arda L. (eds) *Handbook of the Arts in Qualitative Research: Perspectives, Methodologies, Examples, and Issues* pp. 71–82. Thousand Oaks, CA: Sage.

Finney, Brian (1998) Tall tales and brief lives: Angela Carter's *Night at the Circus.* Long Beach, CA: California State University. www.csulb.edu/~bhfinney/carter.html.

Fonow, Mary Margaret and Cook, Judith A. (2005) Feminist methodology: New applications in the academy and public policy. *Signs* 30 (4): 2211–2236.

Foster, Victoria (2007) The art of empathy: Employing the arts in social inquiry with poor working-class women. *Social Justice* 34 (1): 361–376.

Foster, Victoria (2009) Authentic representation? Using video as counter-hegemony in participatory research with poor working-class women. *International Journal of Research Approaches* 3 (3): 233–245.

Foster, Victoria (2012a) The pleasure principle: Employing arts-based methods in social work research. *The European Journal of Social Work* 15 (4): 532–545.

Foster, Victoria (2012b) What if? The use of poetry to promote social justice. *Social Work Education* 31 (6): 742–755.

Foster, Victoria (2013) Pantomime and politics: The story of a performance ethnography. *Qualitative Research* 13 (1): 36–52.

Foster, Victoria (2015) Myths and monsters: Challenging assumptions of poor working class motherhood through feminist research. In Wahab, Stephanie, Anderson-Nathe, Ben and Gringeri, Christina (eds) *Feminisms in Social Work Research* pp. 120–134. Abingdon: Routledge.

Foster, Victoria and Young, Alys (2012) The use of routinely collected health data for research: A critical review. *Health: An Interdisciplinary Journal for the Social Study of Health, Illness and Medicine* 16 (4): 448–463.

Foster, Victoria and Young, Alys (2015) Reflecting on participatory methodologies: Research with parents of babies requiring neonatal care. *International Journal of Social Research Methodology* 18 (1): 91–104.

Foucault, Michel (1977) *Discipline and Punish: The Birth of the Prison.* Translated by Alan Sheridan. London: Penguin. First published in French in 1975 as *Surveiller et Punir*, Paris: Gallimard.

Foucault, Michel (1980) *Power/Knowledge: Selected Interviews and Other Writings, 1972–1977,* translated and edited by Colin Gordon. New York: Pantheon.

Frank, Arthur (1995) *The Wounded Storyteller: Body, Illness and Ethics.* Chicago: University of Chicago Press.

Frank, Arthur W. (2010) *Letting Stories Breathe: A Socio-Narratology.* Chicago: University of Chicago Press.

Frank, Arthur W. (2012) Practicing dialogical narrative analysis. In Holstein, James A. and Gubrium, Jaber F., *Varieties of Narrative Analysis* pp. 33–52. Thousand Oaks, CA: Sage.

Franklin, Ralph W. (1998) *The Poems of Emily Dickinson: Reading Edition.* Cambridge, MA: Belknap Press.

Freeman, Melissa (2011) Validity in dialogic encounters with hermeneutic truths. *Qualitative Inquiry* 17 (6): 543–551.

Freire, Paulo (1970) *Pedagogy of the Oppressed.* New York: Continuum International.

Freire, Paulo and Shor, Ira (1987) *A Pedagogy for Liberation: Dialogues on Transforming Education.* London: Macmillan Education.

Fremeaux, Isabelle and Ramsden, Hilary (2007) We disobey to love: Rebel clowning for social justice. In Clover, Darlene E. and Stalker, Joyce (eds) *The Arts and Social Justice: Re-crafting Adult Education and Community Cultural Leadership* pp. 21–38. Leicester: NIACE.

Fuentes, Carlos (1992) *The Campaign.* New York: Harper Perennial.

Furman, Rich, Langer, C. L., Davis, Christine S., Gallardo, Heather P. and Kilkarni, Shanti (2007) Expressive, research and reflective poetry as qualitative inquiry: A study of adolescent identity. *Qualitative Research* 7 (3): 301–315.

Gardiner, Michael (1992) Bakhtin's carnival: Utopia as critique. *Utopian Studies* 3 (2): 21–49.

Gergen, Mary M. and Gergen, Kenneth J. (2010) Performative social science and psychology. *Forum Qualitative Sozialforschung/Forum: Qualitative Social Research* 12(1): Art. 11, http://nbnresolving.de/urn:nbn:de:0114-fqs1101119.

Gillies, Val and Alldred, Pam (2002) The ethics of intention: Using research as a political tool. In Mauthner, Melanie, Birch, Maxine, Jessop, Julie and Miller, Tina (eds) *Ethics in Qualitative Research* pp. 32–52. London: Sage.

Gordon-Nesbitt, Rebecca (2015) *Exploring the Longitudinal Relationship between Arts Engagement and Health*. Manchester: Arts for Health, Manchester Metropolitan University.

Gramsci, Antonio (1971) *Selections from the Prison Notebooks*. London: Lawrence and Wishart.

Gray, Mel and Schubert, Leanne (2010) Turning base metal into gold: Transmuting art, practice, research and experience into knowledge. *British Journal of Social Work* 40 (7): 2308–2325.

Gray, Ross E. (2003) Performing on and off the stage: The place(s) of performance in arts-based approaches to qualitative inquiry. *Qualitative Inquiry* 9 (2): 254–267.

Greco, Monica and Stenner, Paul (2008) *Emotions: A Social Science Reader*. Abingdon: Routledge.

Greene, Maxine (2000) *Releasing the Imagination: Essays on Education, the Arts, and Social Change*. San Francisco: Jossey-Bass.

Grehan, Helena (2009) *Performance, Ethics and Spectatorship in a Global Age*. Basingstoke: Palgrave Macmillan.

Grenz, Sabine (2005) Intersections of sex and power in research on prostitution: A female researcher interviewing male heterosexual clients. *Signs* 30 (4): 2091–2113.

Gunaratnam, Yasmin (2009) Where is the love? Art, aesthetics and research. In Chamberlayne, Prue and Smith, Martin (eds) *Art, Creativity and Imagination in Social Work Practice* pp. 13–30. Abingdon: Routledge.

Haaken, Janice K. and O'Neill, Maggie (2014) Moving images: Psychoanalytically informed visual methods in documenting the lives of women migrants and asylum seekers. *Journal of Health Psychology* 19 (1): 79–89.

Haffenden, John (1985) *Novelists in Interview*. London: Methuen.

Hafford-Letchfield, Trish, Couchman, Wendy, Webster, Maxine and Avery, Peter (2010) A drama project about older people's intimacy and sexuality. *Educational Gerontology* 36 (7): 604–621.

Hall, Budd L. (2001) I wish this were a poem of practices of participatory research. In Reason, Peter and Bradbury, Hilary (eds) *Handbook of Action Research* pp. 171–178. London: Sage.

Haraway, Donna (1988) Situated knowledges: The science question in feminism and the privilege of partial perspectives. *Feminist Studies* 14 (3): 575–599.

Haraway, Donna (1991) Situated knowledges. In *Simians, Cyborgs, and Women: The Reinvention of Nature* pp. 183–201. New York: Routledge.

Harding, Sandra (1987) *Feminism and Methodology*. Milton Keynes: Open University Press.

Harper, Douglas (2002) Talking about pictures: A case for photo-elicitation. *Visual Studies* 17 (1): 13–26.

Haskins, Ron and Baron, Jon (2011) Building the connection between policy and evidence: The Obama evidence-based initiatives. London: NESTA (National Endowment for Science, Technology and the Arts).

Hawkins, Anne Hunsaker (1998) *Reconstructing Illness: Studies in Pathography*, 2nd revised edn. West Lafayette, IN: Purdue University Press.

Highmore, Ben (2002a) *Everyday Life and Cultural Theory: An Introduction*. Abingdon: Routledge.

Highmore, Ben (ed.) (2002b) *The Everyday Life Reader*. Abingdon: Routledge.

Highmore, Ben (2005) Unprocessed data: Everyday life in the singular. In Harrison, Ellie, Waters, Jim and Jones, Helen (eds) *Day-to-Day Data*. Nottingham: Angel Row Gallery.

Hodges, Caroline E. M., Fenge, Lee-Ann and Cutts, Wendy (2014) Challenging perceptions of disability through performance poetry methods: The 'Seen but Seldom Heard' project. *Disability and Society* 29 (7): 1090–1103.

hooks, bel (1984) *Feminist Theory: From Margin to Center*. Cambridge, MA: South End Press.

Hughes, Jenny with Ruding, Simon (2009) Made to measure? A critical interrogation of applied theatre as intervention with young offenders in the UK. In Prentki, Tim and Preston, Sheila (eds) *The Applied Theatre Reader* pp. 217–225. Abingdon: Routledge.

Humphries, Beth (2000) From critical thought to emancipatory action: Contradictory research goals? In Truman, Carole, Mertens, Donna M. and Humphries, Beth (eds) *Research and Inequality* pp. 179–190. London: UCL Press.

Humphries, Beth (2008) *Social Work Research for Social Justice*. Basingstoke: Palgrave Macmillan.

Hustedde, Ronald and King, Betty (2002) Rituals: Emotions, community faith in soul and the messiness of life. *Community Development Journal* 37 (4): 338–348.

Hyde, Lewis (2008) *Trickster Makes This World: How Disruptive Imagination Creates Culture*. Edinburgh: Canongate.

Inckle, Kay (2010) Telling tales? Using ethnographic fictions to speak embodied 'truth'. *Qualitative Research* 10 (1): 27–47.

Jaggar, Alison M. (1997) Love and knowledge: Emotion in feminist epistemology. In Kemp, Sandra and Squires, Judith (eds) *Feminisms*. Oxford: Oxford University Press

Janesick, Valerie J. (1998) The dance of qualitative research design: Metaphor, methodolatry, and meaning. In Denzin, Norman K. and Lincoln, Yvonna S. (eds) *Strategies of Qualitative Inquiry* pp. 35–55. Thousand Oaks, CA: Sage.

Jay, Gregory S. (2007) Other people's holocausts: Trauma, empathy, and justice in Anna Deavere Smith's *Fires in the Mirror*. *Contemporary Literature* 48 (1): 119–150.

Jenoure, Terry (2008) Hearing Jesua's laugh. In Cahnmann-Taylor, Melisa and Siegesmund, Richard (eds) *Arts-Based Research in Education* pp. 153–181. New York: Routledge.

Jones, Chris and Novak, Tony (1999) *Poverty, Welfare and the Disciplinary State*. London: Routledge.

Jones, Kip (2006a) The art of collaborative storytelling: A discussion on arts-based representations of narrative contexts. In Milnes, Kate, Horrocks, Christine, Kelly, Nancy, Roberts, Brian and Robinson, David (eds) *Narrative, Memory and Knowledge: Representations, Aesthetics and Contexts* pp. 185–196. Huddersfield: University of Huddersfield Press.

Jones, Kip (2006b) A biographic researcher in pursuit of an aesthetic: The use of arts-based (re)presentations in 'performative' dissemination of life stories. *Qualitative Sociology Review* 2 (1): 66–85.

Jones, Omi Osun Joni L. (2002) Performance ethnography: The role of embodiment in cultural authenticity. *Theatre Topics* 12 (1): 1–15.

Jones, Omi Osun Joni L. (2006) Part V introduction: Performance and ethnography, performing ethnography, performance ethnography. In Madison, D. Soyini and Hamera, Judith (eds) *The Sage Handbook of Performance Studies* pp. 339–346. Thousand Oaks, CA: Sage.

Jones, Steve (2006) *Antonio Gramsci*. Abingdon: Routledge.

Kaprow, Allan (2003) *Essays on the Blurring of Art and Life*. Expanded edn. Berkeley and Los Angeles: University of California Press.

Kay, Lisa (2013) Bead collage: An arts-based research method. *International Journal of Education and the Arts* 14 (3): 1–18. www.ijea.org/v14n3/.

Kemmis, Stephen (2001) Exploring the relevance of critical theory for action research: Emancipatory action research in the footsteps of Jürgen Habermas. In Reason, Peter and Bradbury, Hilary (eds) *Handbook of Action Research* pp. 91–102. London: Sage.

Kemp, Amanda (1998) This black body in question. In Phelan, Peggy and Lane, Jill (eds) *The Ends of Performance*. New York: New York University Press.

Kester, Grant H. (2004) *Conversation Pieces: Community and Communication in Modern Art*. Berkeley and Los Angeles: University of California Press.

Kester, Grant H. (2011) *The One and the Many: Contemporary Collaborative Art in a Global Context*. Durham, NC and London: Duke University Press.

Knowles, J. Gary and Thomas, Suzanne M. (2002). Artistry, inquiry, and sense-of-place: Secondary school students portrayed in context. In Bagley, Carl and Cancienne, Mary Beth (eds) *Dancing the Data* pp. 121–132. New York: Peter Lang.

Kothari, Uma (2001) Power, knowledge and social control in participatory development. In Cooke, Bill and Kothari, Uma (eds) *Participation: The New Tyranny* pp. 139–152. London: Zed Books.

Kovach, Margaret (2009) *Indigenous Methodologies: Characteristics, Conversations and Contexts*. Toronto: University of Toronto Press.

Kusserow, Adrie (2008) Ethnographic poetry. In Cahnmann-Taylor, Melisa and Siegesmund, Richard (eds) *Arts-Based Research in Education* pp. 72–78. New York: Routledge.

Kwon, Miwon (2004) *One Place After Another*. Cambridge, MA: MIT Press.

Lacy, Suzanne (2010) *Leaving Art: Writings on Performance, Poetics, and Publics, 1974–2007*. Durham, NC and London: Duke University Press.

Lafrenière, Darquise and Cox, Susan M. (2013) 'If you can call it a poem': Toward a framework for the assessment of arts-based works. *Qualitative Research* 13 (3): 318–336.

Langellier, Kristin M. and Peterson, Eric E. (2004) *Storytelling in Everyday Life: Performing Narrative*. Philadelphia: Temple University Press.

Lapum, Jennifer L., Liu, Linda, Church, Kathryn, Yau, Terrence M., Ruttonsha, Perin, Matthews David, Alison and Retta, Bruk (2014) Arts-informed research dissemination in the health sciences: An evaluation of people's responses to 'The 7,024th Patient' art installation. *Sage Open* 4 (January–March): 1–14.

Lapum, Jennifer, Ruttonsha, Perin, Church, Kathryn, Yau, Terrence and Matthews David, Alison (2012) Employing the arts in research as an analytical tool and dissemination method: Interpreting experience through the aesthetic. *Qualitative Inquiry* 18 (1): 100–115.

Lather, Patti (1991) *Getting Smart: Feminist Research and Pedagogy with/in the Postmodern*. New York: Routledge.

Lather, Patti (2007) *Getting Lost: Feminist Efforts Towards a Double(d) Science*. Albany: State University of New York Press.

Lather, Patti (2010) *Engaging Science Policy: From the Side of the Messy*. New York: Peter Lang.

Lather, Patti (2012) The ruins of neo-liberalism and the construction of a new (scientific) subjectivity. *Cultural Studies of Science Education* 7: 1021–1025.

Latimer, Joanna and Skeggs, Beverley (2011) The politics of imagination: Keeping open and critical. *The Sociological Review* 59 (3): 393–410.

Lather, Patti and Smithies, Chris (1997) *Troubling the Angels: Women Living With HIV/AIDS*. Boulder, CO: Westview Press.

Law, John (2004) *After Method: Mess in Social Science Research*. Abingdon: Routledge.

Lawler, Stephanie (2005) Disgusted subjects: The making of middle-class identities. *The Sociological Review* 53 (3): 429–446.

Leavy, Patricia (2009) *Method Meets Art: Arts-Based Research Practice*. New York: Guilford Press.

Ledwith, M. (2001). Community work as critical pedagogy: Re-inventing Freire and Gramsci. *Community Development Journal* 36 (3): 171–182.

Ledwith, Margaret (2009) Antonio Gramsci and feminism: The elusive nature of power. *Educational Philosophy and Theory* 41 (6): 684–697.

Ledwith, Margaret (2011) *Community Development: A Critical Approach* 2nd edn. Bristol: Policy Press.

Ledwith, Margaret and Springett, Jane (2010) *Participatory Practice: Community-based Action for Transformative Change*. Bristol: Policy Press.

Leggo, Carl (2008) Astonishing silence: Knowing in poetry. In Knowles, J. Gary and Cole, Arda L. (eds) *Handbook of the Arts in Qualitative Research: Perspectives, Methodologies, Examples, and Issues* pp. 165–174, Thousand Oaks, CA: Sage.

Lehmann, Hans-Thies (2006) *Postdramatic Theatre*. Trans: Jürs-Munby, Karen. Abingdon: Routledge.

Leotti, Sandra M. and Muthanna, Jennifer S. (2015) Troubling the binary: A critical look at the dualistic construction of quantitative/qualitative methods in feminist social work research. In Wahab, Stéphanie, Anderson-Nathe, Ben and Gringeri, Christina (eds) *Feminisms in Social Work Research* pp. 170–186. Abingdon: Routledge.

Lev-Aladgem, Shulamith (2000) Carnivalesque enactment at the Children's Medical Centre of Rabin Hospital. *Research in Drama Education* 5 (2): 163–174.

Levitas, Ruth (2004) Let's hear it for Humpty: Social exclusion, the Third Way and cultural capital. *Cultural Trends* 13 (2): 41–56.

Levitas, Ruth (2005) *The Inclusive Society? Social Exclusion and New Labour*. Basingstoke: Palgrave Macmillan.

Lochead, Liz (2003) *Dreaming Frankenstein and Collected Poems 1967–1984*. Edinburgh: Polygon Books.

Lorde, Audre (2000) *Uses of the Erotic: The Erotic as Power*. Tucson, AZ: Kore Press.

Lynch, Kathleen (2000) The role of emancipatory research in the academy. In Byrne, Anne and Lentin, Ronit (eds) *(Re)searching Women: Feminist Research Methodologies in the Social Sciences in Ireland* pp. 73–104. Dublin: Institute of Public Administration.

Lyons, Kristina (2008) Understanding and writing the world. In Cahnmann-Taylor, Melisa and Siegesmund, Richard (eds) *Arts-Based Research in Education* pp. 79–82. New York: Routledge.

MacLure, Maggie (2009) Broken voices, dirty words: On the productive insufficiency of voice. In Jackson, Alicia Youngblood and Mazzei, Lisa A. (eds) *Voice in Qualitative Inquiry* pp. 97–114. Abingdon: Routledge.

Maguire, Patricia (1996) Proposing a more feminist participatory research: Knowing and being embraced openly. In De Koning, Korrie and Martin, Marion (eds) *Participatory Research in Health: Issues and Experiences* pp. 27–39. London: Zed Books.

Maguire, Patricia (2001) Uneven ground: Feminisms and action research. In Reason, Peter and Bradbury, Hilary (eds) *Handbook of Action Research* pp. 59–69. London: Sage.

Malcolm, Janet (2004) *Reading Chekhov: A Critical Journey*. London: Granta Books.

Marsh, Barbara (2003) Wall. In Schneider, Myra, Wood, Dilys and Coles, Gladys Mary (eds) *Making Worlds: One Hundred Contemporary Women Poets*. West Kirkby: Headland Publications.

Marston, Greg and Watts, Rob (2003) Tampering with the evidence: A critical appraisal of evidence-based policy-making. *The Drawing Board: An Australian Review of Public Affairs* 3 (3): 143–163.

Martin, Paul 'Pablo' and Renegar, Valerie (2007) 'The Man for His Time': *The Big Lebowski* as carnivalesque social critique. *Communication Studies* 58 (3): 299–313.

Matarasso, François (1997) *Use or Ornament? The Social Impact of Participation in the Arts*. Stroud: Comedia.

Mattingly, Cheryl and Garro, Linda C. (eds) (2000) *Narrative and the Cultural Construction of Illness and Healing*. Berkeley: University of California Press.

Mazzei, Lisa A. (2009) An impossibly full voice. In Jackson, Alicia Youngblood and Mazzei, Lisa A. (eds) *Voice in Qualitative Inquiry* pp. 45–62. Abingdon: Routledge.

Mazzei, Lisa A. and Jackson, Alicia Youngblood (2009) Introduction: The limits of voice. In Jackson, Alicia Youngblood and Mazzei, Lisa A. (eds) *Voice in Qualitative Inquiry* pp. 1–14. Abingdon: Routledge.

McLaren, Peter (1999) Foreword. In Shapiro, Sherry, *Pedagogy and the Politics of the Body: A Critical Praxis* pp. viii–xvi. New York: Garland.

McLaughlin, Hugh (2006) Involving young service users as co-researchers: Possibilities, benefits and costs. *British Journal of Social Work* 36: 1395–1410.

McNiff, Shaun (1998) *Arts-Based Research*. London: Jessica Kingsley.

McRobbie, Angela (2001) 'Everyone is creative': Artists as pioneers of the new economy? *Open Democracy*. www.opendemocracy.net/node/652.

Mengham, Ron (2001) Bourgeois news: Humphrey Jennings and Charles Madge. *New Formations* no. 44 (Autumn): 26–33.

Mey, Kerstin (2010) Afterword: In/ter/ceptions and in/tensions – Situating Suzanne Lacy's practice. In Lacy, Suzanne, *Leaving Art: Writings on Performance, Poetics, and Publics, 1974–2007* pp. 327–338. Durham, NC and London: Duke University Press.

Mienczakowski, Jim (1996) An ethnographic act: The construction of consensual theatre. In Ellis, Carolyn and Bochner, Arthur P. (eds) *Composing Ethnography: Alternative Forms of Qualitative Writing* pp. 244–264. Walnut Creek, CA: AltaMira Press.

Mienczakowski, Jim (2000) Ethnography in the form of theatre with emancipatory intentions. In Truman, Carole, Mertens, Donna M. and Humphries, Beth (eds) *Research and Inequality* pp. 126–142. London: UCL Press.

Mienczakowski, Jim and Morgan, Stephen (2001) Ethnodrama: Constructing participatory, experiential and compelling action research through performance. In Reason, Peter and Bradbury, Hilary (eds) *Handbook of Action Research* pp. 219–227. London: Sage.

Mies, Maria (1983) Towards a methodology for feminist research. In Bowles, Gloria and Duelli Klein, Renate (eds) *Theories of Women's Studies*. London: Routledge and Kegan Paul.

Mitchell, W. J. T. (2002) Showing seeing: A critique of visual culture. *Journal of Visual Culture* 1 (2): 165–181.

Mohanty, Chandra Talpade (1984) Under Western eyes: Feminist scholarship and colonial discourses. *Boundary 2* 12 (3): 333–358.

Murdoch, Iris (1999) *The Black Prince*. London: Vintage.

Nicholson, Helen (2005) *Applied Drama: The Gift of Theatre*. Basingstoke: Palgrave Macmillan.

Nogueira, Marcia Pompeo, Gonçalves, Reonaldo Manoel and Prentki, Tim (2014) Between popular traditions and forum theatre: Playing on the borders of Theatre of the Oppressed. *Applied Theatre Research* 2 (2): 183–195.

Oakley, Ann (1992) *Social Support and Motherhood*. Oxford: Blackwell.

O'Connor, Deborah L. and O'Neill, Brian J. (2004) Toward social justice. *Journal of Teaching in Social Work* 24 (3–4): 19–33.

O'Neill, Maggie (2008) Transnational refugees: The transformative role of art? *Forum Qualitative Sozialforschung/Forum: Qualitative Social Research* 9 (2): Art. 59, http://nbn-resolving.de/urn:nbn:de:0114–fqs0802590.

O'Neill, Maggie with Giddens, Sara, Breatnach, Patricia, Bagley, Carl, Bourne, Darren and Judge, Tony (2002) Renewed methodologies for social research: Ethno-mimesis as performative praxis. *The Sociological Review* 50 (1): 69–88.

Osler and Zhu (2011) Narratives in teaching and research for justice and human rights. *Education, Citizenship and Social Justice* 6 (3): 223–235.

Packard, Josh (2008) 'I'm gonna show you what it's really like out here': The power and limitation of participatory visual methods. *Visual Studies* 23 (1): 63–77.

Pariser, David (2009) Arts-based research: Trojan horses and shibboleths. The liabilities of a hybrid research approach. What hath Eisner wrought? *Canadian Review of Art Education* 36 (1): 1–18.

Parker-Starbuck, Jennifer and Moch, Roberta (2012) Researching the body in/as performance. In Kershaw, Baz and Nicholson, Helen (eds) *Research Methods in Theatre and Performance* pp. 210–235. Edinburgh: Edinburgh University Press.

Pease, Bob (2002) Rethinking empowerment: A postmodern reappraisal for emancipatory practice. *British Journal of Social Work* 32 (2): 135–147.

Pechey, Graham (2007) *Mikhail Bakhtin: The Word in the World*. London: Routledge.

Pelias, Ronald J. (2008) Performative inquiry: Embodiment and its challenges. In Knowles, J. Gary and Cole, Ardra L. (eds) *Handbook of the Arts in Qualitative Research: Perspectives, Methodologies, Examples, and Issues* pp. 186–195. Thousand Oaks, CA: Sage.

Perec, Georges (2008) *Species of Space and Other Pieces*. London: Penguin Classics.

Piirto, Jane (2002) The question of quality and qualifications: Writing inferior poems as qualitative research. *International Journal of Qualitative Studies in Education* 15 (4): 431–445.

Pink, Sarah (2007) *Doing Visual Ethnography*, 2nd edn. London: Sage.

Plummer, Ken (1995) *Telling Sexual Stories: Power, Change and Social Worlds*. London: Routledge.

Ponic, Pamela and Jategaonkar, Natasha (2012) Balancing safety and action: Ethical protocols for photovoice research with women who have experienced violence. *Arts* and Health: An International Journal for Research, Policy and Practice 4 (3): 189–202.

Popay, Jennie, Thomas, Carol, Williams, Gareth, Bennett, Sharon, Gatrell, Anthony and Bostock, Lisa (2003) A proper place to live: Health inequalities, agency and the normative dimensions of space. *Social Science and Medicine* 57 (1): 55–69.

Prendergast, Monica (2009) Introduction: The phenomena of poetry in research: 'Poem is What?' Poetic inquiry in qualitative social science research. In Prendergast, Monica, Leggo, Carl and Sameshima, Pauline (eds) *Poetic Inquiry: Vibrant Voices in the Social Sciences* pp. xix–xlii. Rotterdam: Sense Publishers.

Prentki, Tim (2006) Conversations with the Devil. *Applied Theatre Researcher/IDEA Journal* 7: 1–11.

Prentki, Tim (2009a) Introduction to poetics of representation. In Prentki, Tim and Preston, Sheila (eds) *The Applied Theatre Reader* pp. 19–21. Abingdon: Routledge.

Prentki, Tim (2009b) Applied theatre in a global village. In Prentki, Tim and Preston, Sheila (eds) *The Applied Theatre Reader* pp. 363–367. Abingdon: Routledge.

Prentki, Tim (2012) *The Fool in EuropeanTheatre: Stages of Folly*. Basingstoke: Palgrave Macmillan.

Prentki, Tim and Preston, Sheila (2009) Applied theatre: An introduction. In Prentki, Tim and Preston, Sheila (eds) *The Applied Theatre Reader* pp. 9–16. Abingdon: Routledge.

Preston, Sheila (2009a) Introduction to ethics of representation. In Prentki, Tim and Preston, Sheila (eds) *The Applied Theatre Reader* pp. 65–69. Abingdon: Routledge.

Preston, Sheila (2009b) Introduction to transformation. In Prentki, Tim and Preston, Sheila (eds) *The Applied Theatre Reader* pp. 303–306. Abingdon: Routledge.

Quinney, Richard (1998) *For the Time Being: Ethnography of Everyday Life*. Albany: State University of New York Press.

Rankin, Lissa (2015) *The Fear Cure: Cultivating Courage as Medicine for the Body, Mind and Soul*. London: Hay House.

Rasberry G. W. (2002) Imagine: Inventing a data-dancer. In Bagley, Carl and Cancienne, Mary Beth (eds) *Dancing the Data* pp. 105–120. New York: Peter Lang.

Rath, Jean (2012). Poetry and participation: Scripting a meaningful research text with rape crisis worker. *Forum Qualitative Sozialforschung/Forum: Qualitative Social Research* 13(1): Art. 22, http://nbn-resolving.de/urn:nbn:de:0114–fqs1201224.

Ravenscroft, Neil and Gilchrist, Paul (2009) Spaces of transgression: Governance, discipline and reworking the carnivalesque. *Leisure Studies* 28 (1): 35–49.

Reason, Peter (1998) Three approaches to participative inquiry. In Denzin, Norman K. and Lincoln, Yvonna S. (eds) *Strategies of Qualitative Inquiry* pp. 261–291. Thousand Oaks, CA: Sage

Reason, Peter (2000) Action research as spiritual practice. Learning Community Conference, University of Surrey, UK, 4–5 May.

Reason, Peter and Bradbury, Hilary (eds) (2001) *Handbook of Action Research: Participative Inquiry and Practice*. London: Sage.

Reason, Peter and Rowan, John (eds) (1981) *Human Inquiry: A Sourcebook of New Paradigm Research*. Chichester: Wiley.

Rhodes, Colin (2000) *Outsider Art: Spontaneous Alternatives*. London: Thames and Hudson.

Richardson, Jack (2010) Interventionist art education: Contingent communities, social dialogue, and public collaboration. *Studies in Art Education* 52(1): 18–33.

Richardson, Laurel (1990a) Narrative and sociology. *Journal of Contemporary Ethnography* 19 (1): 116–135.

Richardson, Laurel (1990b) *Writing Strategies: Reaching Diverse Audiences.* Newbury Park, CA: Sage.

Richardson, Laurel (1998) Writing: A method of inquiry. In Denzin, Norman K. and Lincoln, Yvonna S. (eds) *Collecting and Interpreting Qualitative Materials.* Thousand Oaks, CA: Sage.

Riggio, Milla Cozart (2004a) Time out or time in? The urban dialectic of carnival. In Riggio, Milla Cozart (ed.) *Carnival: Culture in Action – The Trinidad Experience* pp. 13–30. Abingdon: Routledge.

Riggio, Milla Cozart (2004b) The carnival story – then and now: Introduction to Part I. In Riggio, Milla Cozart (ed.) *Carnival: Culture in Action – The Trinidad Experience* pp. 39–47. Abingdon: Routledge.

Roth, Moira (2001) Making and Performing Code 33: A public art project with Suzanne Lacy, Julio Morales, and Unique Holland. *PAJ: A Journal of Performance and Art* 23 (3): 47–62.

Roth, Moira (2010) Introduction: Suzanne Lacy – Three decades of performing and writing/writing and performing. In Lacy, Suzanne *Writings on Performance, Politics and Publics, 1974–2007* pp. xvii–xli. Durham, NC and London: Duke University Press.

RSPH (Royal Society for Public Health) (2013) *Arts, Health and Wellbeing Beyond the Millennium: How Far Have We Come and Where Do We Want to Go?* London: RSPH and the Philipp Family Foundation.

Rule, Peter (2004) Dialogic spaces: Adult education projects and social engagement. *International Journal of Lifelong Education* 23 (4): 319–334.

Saldaña, Johnny (2008) Ethnodrama and ethnotheatre. In Knowles, J. Gary and Cole, Ardra L. (eds) *Handbook of the Arts in Qualitative Research: Perspectives, Methodologies, Examples, and Issues* pp. 195–207. Thousand Oaks, CA: Sage.

Saldaña, Johnny (2011) *Ethnotheatre: Research from Page to Stage.* Walnut Creek, CA: Left Coast Press.

Saldaña, Johnny, Finley, Susan and Finley, Macklin (2005) Street rat. In Saldaña, Johnny, *Ethnodrama: An Anthology of Reality Theatre* pp. 139– 179. Walnut Creek, CA: Alta Mira Press.

Salverson, Julie (2001) Change on whose terms? Testimony and an erotics of inquiry. *Theater* 31 (3): 119–125.

Sandelowski, Margarete (1994) The proof is in the pottery: Toward a poetic for qualitative inquiry. In Morse, Janice M. (ed.) *Critical Issues in Qualitative Research Methods* pp. 46–63. Thousand Oaks, CA: Sage.

Saunders, Gill (2010) How wallpaper left home and made an exhibition of itself. In Saunders, Gill (ed.) *Walls are Talking: Wallpaper, Art and Culture* pp. 27–95. Manchester: Whitworth Art Gallery.

Schechner, Richard (1985) *Between Theatre and Anthropology.* Philadelphia: University of Pennsylvania Press.

Seeley, Chris and Reason, Peter (2008) Expressions of energy: An epistemologicy of presentational knowing. In Liamputtong, Pranee and Rumbold, Jean (eds) *Knowing Differently: Arts-based and Collaborative Research Methods* pp. 25–46. New York: Nova Science.

Servaes, Jan (1996) Introduction: Particiaptory communication and research in development settings. In Servaes, Jan, Jacobson, Thomas L. and White, Shirley A. (eds) *Participatory Communication for Social Change* pp. 13–25. New Delhi: Sage.

Shapiro, Sherry (1999) *Pedagogy and the Politics of the Body: A Critical Praxis.* New York: Garland.

Sharma, Sonya, Reimer-Kirkham, Sheryl and Cochrane, Marie (2009) Practising the awareness of embodiment in qualitative health research: Methodological reflections. *Qualitative Health Research* 19 (11): 1642–1650.

Shepherd, Simon (2006) *Theatre, Body and Pleasure*. Abingdon: Routledge.

Sheringham, Michael (2006) *Everyday Life: Theories and Practices from Surrealism to the Present*. Oxford: Oxford University Press.

Shulz, Christoph Benjamin (2011) Down the rabbit hole and into the museum: Alice and the visual arts. In Delahunty, Gavin and Schulz, Christoph Benjamin (eds) *Alice in Wonderland Through the Visual Arts* pp. 8–35. Liverpool: Tate Liverpool.

Siegesmund, Richard and Cahnmann-Taylor, Melisa (2008) The tensions of arts-based research in education reconsidered: The promise for practice. In Cahnmann-Taylor, Melisa and Siegesmund, Richard (eds) *Arts-Based Research in Education* pp. 231–246. New York: Routledge.

Simons, Helen and McCormack, Brendan (2007) Integrating arts-based inquiry in evaluation methodology: Opportunities and challenges. *Qualitative Inquiry* 13 (2): 292–311.

Singh, Madhu (2009) Weapon of the weak (?): Reading resistance in select short stories by Bangladeshi women writers. *Journal of the School of Language, Literature and Culture Studies*, Jawaharlal Nehru University, New Delhi. Spring: 1–18.

Skeggs, Beverley (1997) *Formations of Class and Gender: Becoming Respectable*. London: Sage.

Skeggs, Beverley (2004) *Class, Self, Culture*. London: Routledge.

Smith, Dorothy (1987) *The Everyday World as Problematic: A Feminist Sociology*. Boston: Northeastern University Press.

Smith, Dorothy (1992) Sociology from women's experience: A reaffirmation. *Sociological Theory* 10 (1): 88–98.

Smith, Linda Tuhiwai (2012) *Decolonizing Methodologies: Research and Indigenous Peoples*, 2nd edn. London: Zed Books.

Smith, Roger (2009) *Doing Social Work Research*. Maidenhead: Open University Press.

Snowber, Celeste (2002) Bodydance: Enfleshing soulful inquiry through improvisation. In Bagley, Carl and Cancienne, Mary Beth (eds) *Dancing the Data* pp. 20–33. New York: Peter Lang.

Snowber, Celeste and Bickel, Barbara (2015) Companions with mystery: Art, spirit and the ecstatic. In Walsh, Susan, Bickel, Barbara and Leggo, Carl (eds) *Arts-based and Contemplative Practices in Research and Teaching* pp. 67–87. New York and Abingdon: Routledge.

Snyder-Young, Dani (2010) Beyond 'An aesthetic of objectivity': Performance ethnography, performance texts, and theatricality. *Qualitative Inquiry* 16 (10): 883–893.

Solomos, John (1998) Series editor's preface. In Bhattacharyya, Gargi, *Tales of Dark-skinned Women: Race, Gender and Global Culture*. London: UCL Press.

Spivak, Gayatri Chakravorty (1987) *In Other Worlds: Essays in Cultural Politics*. New York: Methuen.

St. Pierre, Elizabeth Adams (2009) Afterword: Decentering voice in qualitative inquiry. In Jackson, Alicia Youngblood and Mazzei, Lisa A. (eds) *Voice in Qualitative Inquiry* pp. 221–236. Abingdon: Routledge.

Stacey, Judith (1988) Can there be a feminist ethnography? *Women's Studies International Forum* 11(1): 21–27.

Stanley, Liz (1990) An editorial introduction. In Stanley, Liz (ed.) *Feminist Praxis: Research, Theory and Epistemology in Feminist Sociology* pp. 3–19. London: Routledge.

Starhawk (1987) *Truth or Dare: Encounters with Power, Authority, and Mystery.* New York: Harper and Row.

Szakolczai, Arpad (2007) Image-magic in *A Midsummer Night's Dream*: Power and modernity from Weber to Shakespeare. *History of the Human Sciences* 20 (4): 1–26.

Tate Gallery (2012) *Suzanne Lacy: The Crystal Quilt.* www.tate.org.uk/whats-on/tate-modern-tanks/display/suzanne-lacy-crystal-quilt.

Taylor, Millie (2007) *British Pantomime Performance.* Bristol: Intellect.

Thomas, Robyn and Davies, Annette (2005) What have the feminists done for us? Feminist theory and organizational resistance. *Organization* 12 (5): 711–740.

Thompson, James (2003) *Applied Theatre: Bewilderment and Beyond.* New York: Peter Lang.

Thompson, James (2009) *Performance Affects: Applied Theatre and the End of Effects.* Basingstoke: Palgrave Macmillan.

Thrift, Nigel and Dewsbury, John-David (2000) Dead geographies – and how to make them live. *Environment and Planning D: Society and Space* 18 (4): 411–432.

Tolle, Eckhart (2001) *The Power of Now.* London: Hodder and Stoughton.

Trinh T. Minh-ha (1991) *When the Moon Waxes Red: Representation, Gender and Cultural Politics.* New York: Routledge.

Tyler, Imogen (2008) Chav mum chav scum. *Feminist Media Studies* 8 (1): 17–34.

utalkmarketing.com (2007) Aaaaaah tissue! 4 January. www.utalkmarketing.com/pages/article.aspx?articleid=891&title=aaaaaah_tissue!

Valentine, James (2008) Narrative acts: Telling tales of life and love with the wrong gender. *Forum Qualitative Sozialforschung/Forum: Qualitative Social Research* 9 (2): Art. 49, http://nbn-resolving.de/urn:nbn:de:0114-fqs0802491.

van Son, Romanie (2000) Painting women into the picture. In Byrne, Anne and Lentin, Ronit (eds) *(Re)searching Women: Feminist Research Methodologies in the Social Sciences in Ireland* pp. 214–236. Dublin: Institute of Public Administration.

Visweswaran, Kamala (1994) *Fictions of Feminist Ethnography.* Minneapolis: University of Minnesota Press.

Wahab, Stéphanie, Anderson-Nathe, Ben and Gringeri, Christina (2015) Introduction. In Wahab, Stéphanie, Anderson-Nathe, Ben and Gringeri, Christina (eds) *Feminisms in Social Work Research* pp. 3–15. Abingdon: Routledge.

Walsh, Susan, Bickel, Barbara and Leggo, Carl (2015) *Arts-based and Contemplative Practices in Research and Teaching: Honoring Presence.* New York and Abingdon: Routledge.

Walton, Ginger, Schleien, Stuart J., Brake, Lyndsey R., Trovato, Catherine 'Cat' and Oakes, Tyler (2012) Photovoice: A collaborative methodology giving voice to undeserved populations seeking community inclusion. *Therapeutic Recreation Journal* 46 (3): 168–178.

Wang, Caroline (1999) Photovoice: A participatory action research strategy applied to women's health. *Journal of Women's Health* 8: 185–92.

Warner, Marina (1995) *From the Beast to the Blonde: On Fairy Tales and Their Tellers.* London: Vintage.

Warner, Marina (2000) *No Go The Bogeyman: Scaring, Lulling and Making Mock.* London: Vintage.

Warner, Marina (2011) *Stranger Magic: Charmed States and the Arabian Nights*. London: Chatto and Windus.

Webb, Kate (1994) Seriously funny. In Sage, Lorna (ed.) *Flesh and the Mirror: Essays on the Art of Angela Carter* pp. 279–307. London: Virago Press.

Weitz, Rose (2001) Women and their hair: Seeking power through resistance and accommodation. *Gender and Society* 15 (5): 667–686.

West, Cornel (1993) Foreword. In Deavere Smith, Anna, *Fires in the Mirror*. New York: Anchor Books.

West, Nora and Stalker, Joyce (2007) Journey to a (bi)cultural identity. In Clover, Darlene E. and Stalker, Joyce (eds) *The Arts and Social Justice: Re-crafting Adult Education and Community Cultural Leadership* pp. 125–143. Leicester: NIACE.

Wheeler, Peter (2012) Sightless vision: Reflections on a paradox. *Culture and Organization* 18 (4): 285–304.

Whitmore, Elizabeth (1994) To tell the truth: Working with oppressed groups in participatory approaches to inquiry. In Reason, Peter (ed.) *Participation in Human Inquiry* pp. 82–98. London: Sage.

Wiebe, Sean and Snowber, Celeste (2011) The visceral imagination: A fertile space for non-textual knowing. *Journal of Curriculum Theorizing* 27 (2): 101–113.

Wiles, Rose, Prosser, Jon, Bagnoli, Anna, Clark, Andrew, Davies, Katherine, Holland, Sally and Renold, Emma (2008) Visual ethics: Ethical issues in visual research. ESRC National Centre for Research Methods Review Paper.

Wilkins, Helen (1993) Taking it personally: A note on emotion and autobiography. *Sociology* 27 (1): 93–100.

Willet, John (1977) *The Theatre of Bertolt Brecht*. London: Methuen.

Williams, Fiona (2004) In and beyond New Labour: Towards a new political ethics of care. *Critical Social Policy* 24 (3): 406–427.

Williams, Simon J. (1998) Health as moral performance: Ritual, transgression and taboo. *Health: An Interdisciplinary Journal for the Social Study of Health, Illness and Medicine* 2 (4): 435–457.

Willis, Peter (2008) The work of portrayal: Expressive approaches to educational research. In Liamputtong, Pranee and Rumbold, Jean (eds) *Knowing Differently: Arts-Based and Collaborative Research Methods* pp. 49–65. New York: Nova.

Wiltshire, Kim and Hine, Paul (2014) *Project XXX*. Twickenham: Aurora Metro Publications.

Winston, Joe (2006) Beauty, goodness and education: The Arts beyond utility. *Journal of Moral Education* 35 (3): 285–300.

Winterson, Jeanette (1985) *Oranges Are Not the Only Fruit*. London: Pandora.

Winterson, Jeanette (1996) *Art Objects: Essays on Ecstasy and Effrontery*. London: Vintage.

Witkin Stanley L. (2000) An integrative human rights approach to social research. In Truman, Carole, Mertens, Donna M. and Humphries, Beth (eds) *Research and Inequality* pp. 205–219. London: UCL Press.

Wolff, Janet (1993) *The Social Production of Art*, 2nd edn. Basingstoke: Palgrave Macmillan.

Woods, Christine (2010) Introduction: It's the background that explains the foreground. In Saunders, Gill (ed.) *Walls Are Talking: Wallpaper, Art and Culture* pp. 10–22. Manchester: Whitworth Art Gallery.

Wright Mills, C. (1959) *The Sociological Imagination*. New York: Oxford University Press.

Wulf-Andersen, Trine (2012) Poetic representation: Working with dilemmas of involvement in participative social work research. *European Journal of Social Work* 15 (4): 563–580.

Young-Eisendrath, Polly (1997) *The Resilient Spirit: Transforming Suffering into Insight and Renewal.* Cambridge, MA: Perseus Publishing.

Index

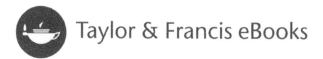

Taylor & Francis eBooks

Helping you to choose the right eBooks for your Library

Add Routledge titles to your library's digital collection today. Taylor and Francis ebooks contains over 50,000 titles in the Humanities, Social Sciences, Behavioural Sciences, Built Environment and Law.

Choose from a range of subject packages or create your own!

Benefits for you

>> Free MARC records
>> COUNTER-compliant usage statistics
>> Flexible purchase and pricing options
>> All titles DRM-free.

Benefits for your user

>> Off-site, anytime access via Athens or referring URL
>> Print or copy pages or chapters
>> Full content search
>> Bookmark, highlight and annotate text
>> Access to thousands of pages of quality research at the click of a button.

REQUEST YOUR FREE INSTITUTIONAL TRIAL TODAY

Free Trials Available
We offer free trials to qualifying academic, corporate and government customers.

eCollections – Choose from over 30 subject eCollections, including:

Archaeology	Language Learning
Architecture	Law
Asian Studies	Literature
Business & Management	Media & Communication
Classical Studies	Middle East Studies
Construction	Music
Creative & Media Arts	Philosophy
Criminology & Criminal Justice	Planning
Economics	Politics
Education	Psychology & Mental Health
Energy	Religion
Engineering	Security
English Language & Linguistics	Social Work
Environment & Sustainability	Sociology
Geography	Sport
Health Studies	Theatre & Performance
History	Tourism, Hospitality & Events

For more information, pricing enquiries or to order a free trial, please contact your local sales team:
www.tandfebooks.com/page/sales

 Routledge
Taylor & Francis Group

The home of
Routledge books

www.tandfebooks.com